Get Fit! For Snowboarding:

I aim to provide you with a useful guide for getting fit for snowboarding, whether you are a seasoned boarder or taking to the slopes for the first time this guide will help you become fitter for the slopes and reduce the risk of injury and aches and pains associated with this sport

Contents

- Introduction

- Pre boarding, pre holiday workout

- Pre boarding, on holiday workout

- Post boarding stretches

Snowboarding is an extremely physical sport, so whether you are taking to the slopes for the first time or a seasoned boarder getting fit and targeting the muscles used in this sport before you go, and during your holiday, is paramount to avoid injury and ease the first few days aches and pains

In the first section we will cover pre holiday training, a programme of strengthening and toning exercises that will get you in peak condition to take in the slopes

In the second section we will focus on your day on the mountain giving you a warm up, pre and post boarding stretches

Cardio training

The simple fact is if you want to be able to make the most out of your holiday and get more runs in you need to start to improve your cardio fitness. This will help you build stamina and strength that will benefit your boarding immensely
You will also find that simple walking at altitude or hiking to get those un-ridden snowfields will be more achievable if your cardio fitness is at a good level

I recommend that you add at least one of the following activities to your weekly workout programme - not just in the build up to your holiday but for all year round, choose an activity that you enjoy so that you will stick you it, or switch them about so you don't get bored of the same thing
You need to do a cardio activity at least 3 times per week.

Running – outdoors or treadmill – minimum 20 minutes per session
Cycling – outdoors and including spinning – minimum 45 minutes
HIIT – check out workouts by Shaun T and Beachbody.com or various on YouTube
– HIIT can be done in just 10 minutes per day – although the ones you can buy from Beachbody.com are 25-50 minutes and very intense!

All of these activities will all improve your cardiovascular system

Complimentary Exercises

Yoga and Pilates are also complementary classes to be adding to your general fitness programme and I will use them in the book to demonstrate specific exercises that benefit the main muscle groups used during snowboarding

Before you go -

Try to start this programme between 4-6 weeks prior to heading to the slopes, if you have less time than that you will still benefit from targeting the muscle groups used up to a week before your trip, any less time than that be prepared to ache and feel tired for the first few days of your holiday!
Ease the aches and re-energise before and after each session on the slopes with the pre and post sections

Warm up

Jogging on the spot timed for 1 min

Jacks – jump in and out on the spot for 1 min

Kick backs - kick the legs behind you so they tap the behind for 30 seconds

High knees – jogging bringing the knees up higher than the waist for 30 seconds

Ski jumps – jump from side to side in a parallel position, using the arms as if you had ski poles for 30 seconds

Repeat - total 8 minutes warm up

A video of this warm up can be found on my YouTube channel the link to it is:
https://www.youtube.com/watch?v=rExKGkr1am4
Or search get fit for snowboarding warm up
Another 7-minute tabata style warm up can be found here:
https://www.youtube.com/watch?v=TOcsR6Not6w&list=UUiNS9wq60MYm_n-cDWrZ5qg
Or check out my blog for more warm up ideas
http://getfitsnow.blogspot.co.uk/

Stretch out after cardio:
Roll down spine to floor, ben knees, and hands flat on floor. Reach back with right foot into lunge, straighten both legs, lower again to lunge, pivot to side, walk through, repeat lunge, straight leg and lunge, pivot back to start, roll back up to standing through the spine, straightening each vertebrae one at a time.

Strengthening exercises

Legs - the quads are the main muscles used both on piste and free riding, therefore strength in quads is important I will focus on building some strength in the quads by using a mixture of strengthening and toning exercises, these positions are all meant to be held for minimum of 30 seconds, or 5 deep in and out breaths. Lots of these exercises are based in Hatha Yoga, so ideally you could find a good Hatha class to be guided through these positions

Wall seat

Try to keep the knees at right angles and hold this position

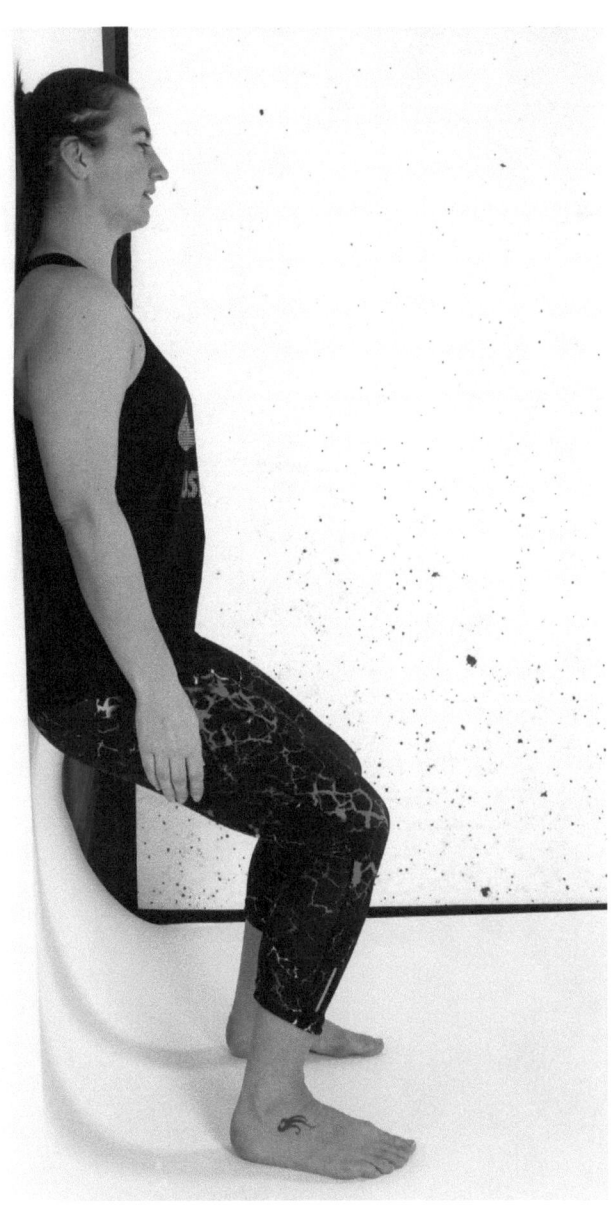

Power Squats

Make sure your knees stay over the toes, to maximize the strength in the quads keep your back straight. You can lower and either hold for 30 seconds or bend and straighten the knees for 1 minute.

Photo of start and finish here

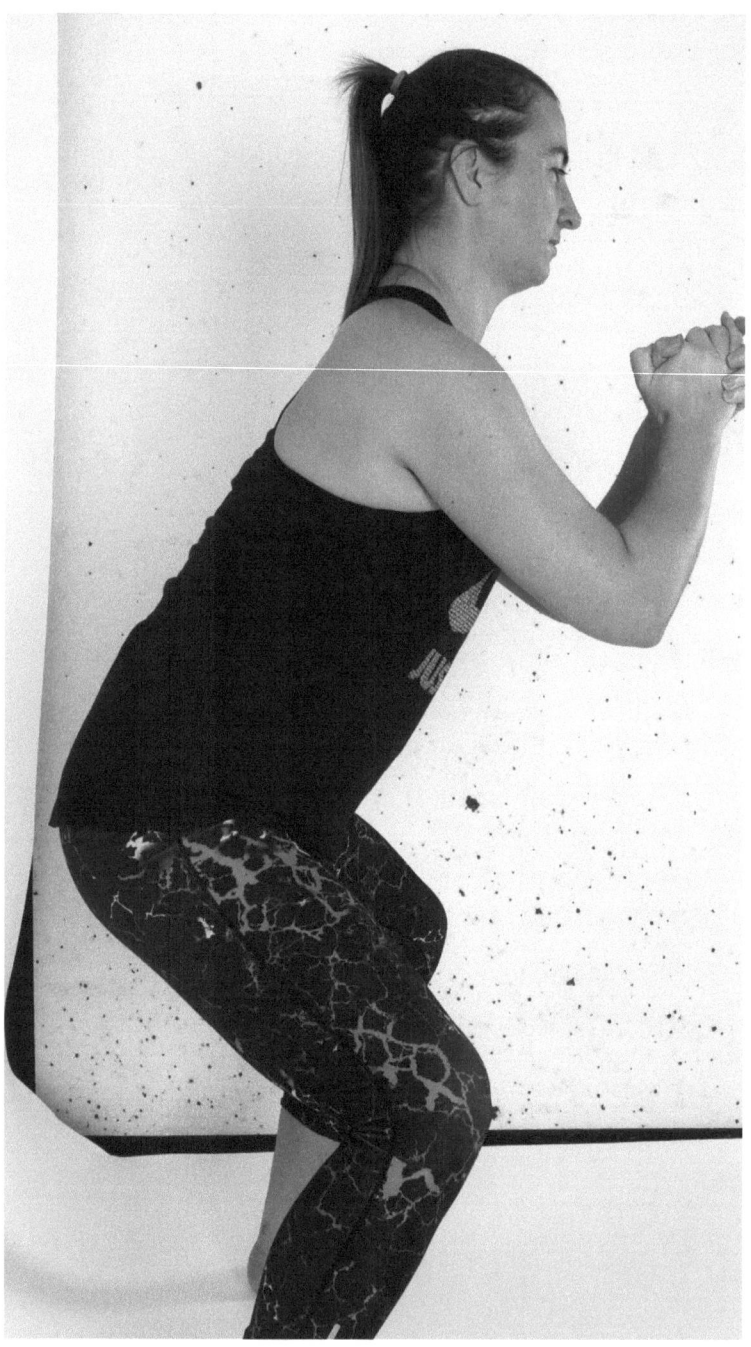

Lunges

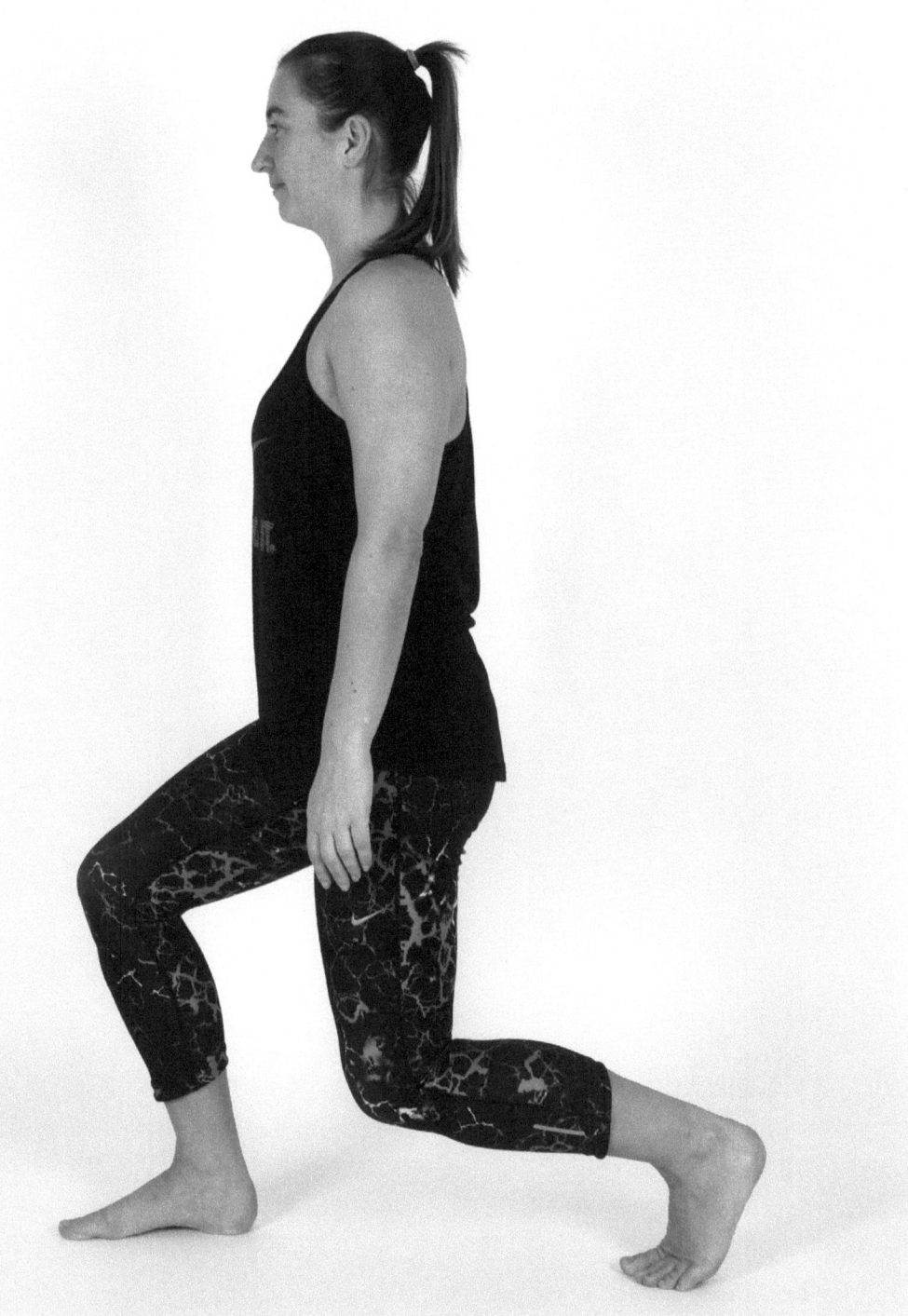

This traditional quad lunge can be done alone or with hand weights, remember to keep right angles in the knees and keep the knees over the toes.

Warrior 1

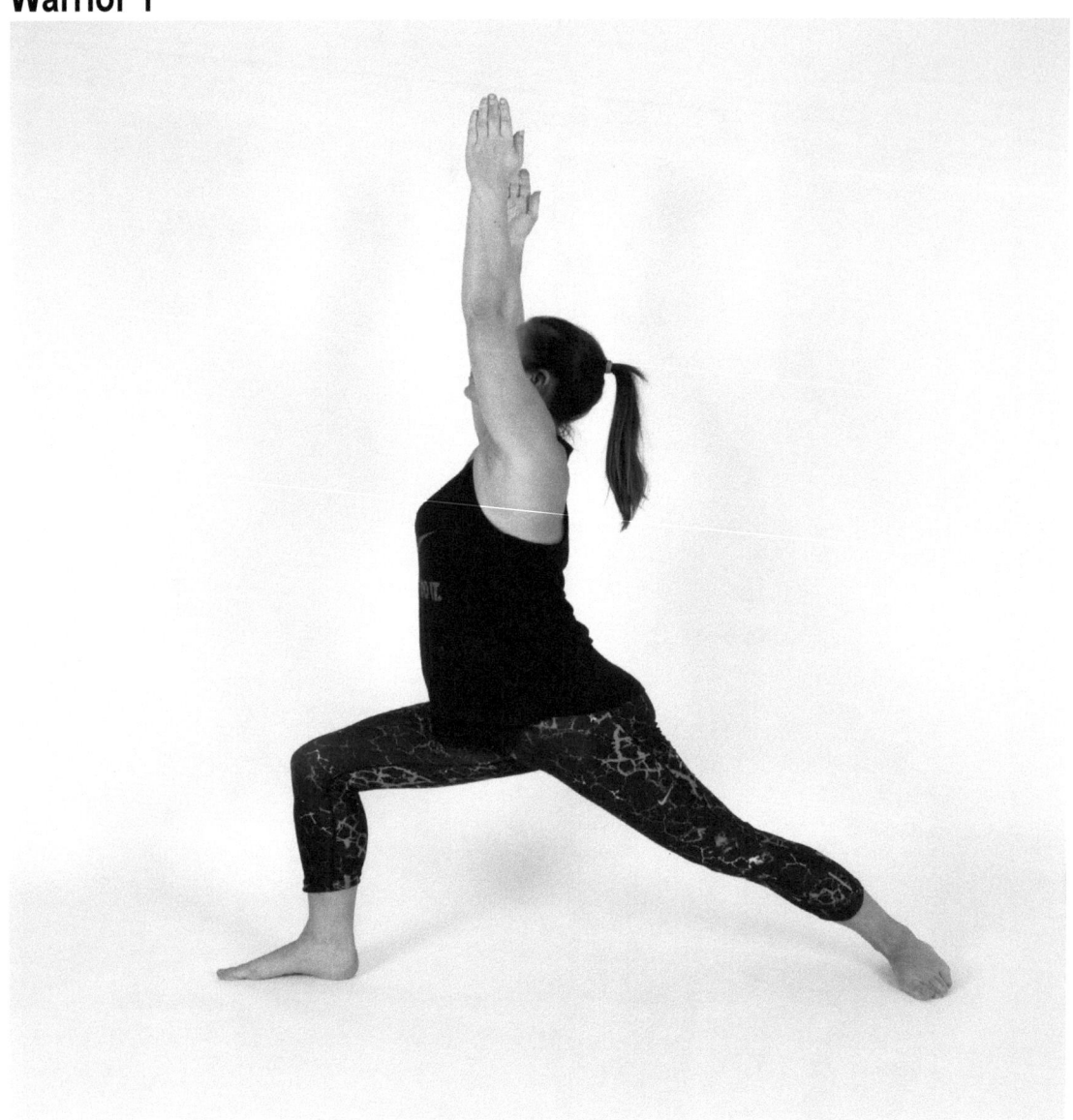

Start with feet together then take the right leg back, pivot the back (right) leg at a 45-degree angle and keep the left foot facing forward. Bend the knee over the front foot, making sure you have knee over toe but that you can still see your foot, do not over stretch this. Raise the arms above the head, in line with your ears.

Hold the stretch for 5, deep in and out breaths. Try to breath through the nose, keeping the mouth closed.

Take the gaze up to the hands if it is comfortable for you

Warrior 2

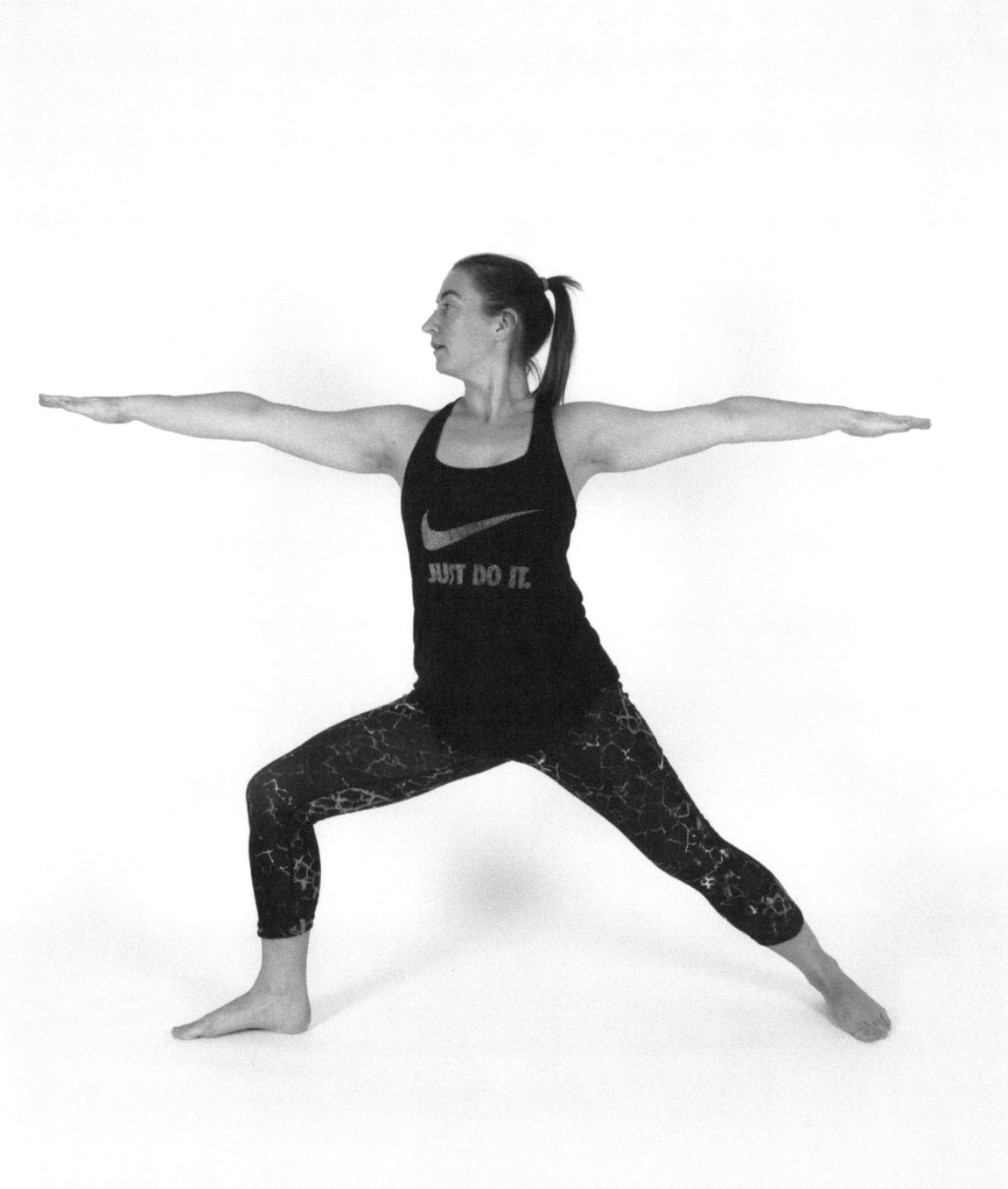

Start with a wide leg stance, then turn out the left (front) foot and turn in the right (back) foot. Bend the knee over the front foot, making sure you have knee over toe but that you can still see your foot, do not over stretch this. Raise the arms to shoulder height and take gaze over the front arm.

Hold the stretch for 5, deep in and out breaths. Try to breath through the nose, keeping the mouth closed

Triangle pose

Start with a wide leg stance, then turn out the left (front) foot and turn in the right (back) foot. Keep both legs straight behind the knee. Bring the arms up to shoulder height, as in Warrior 2, and then reach away from the torso at an angle before you lower the front arm to the toes. Imagine that you are trapped between two panes of glass, so that you keep the top shoulder back and your shoulders are stacked.
Hold the stretch for 5, deep in and out breaths. Try to breath through the nose, keeping the mouth closed

These three yoga 'stretches' are very effective at building strength in the legs.

Upper body - upper body needs to be strong as a lot of the time your run will start from a seated position tightening up your bindings. As a beginner you will need strength in the biceps, triceps and shoulders to push yourselves up after the inevitable falls you may have!

Off piste free riding you will need strength in the arms should the situation arise when you have to be able to dig yourself out of deep snow and powder

Triangle press ups

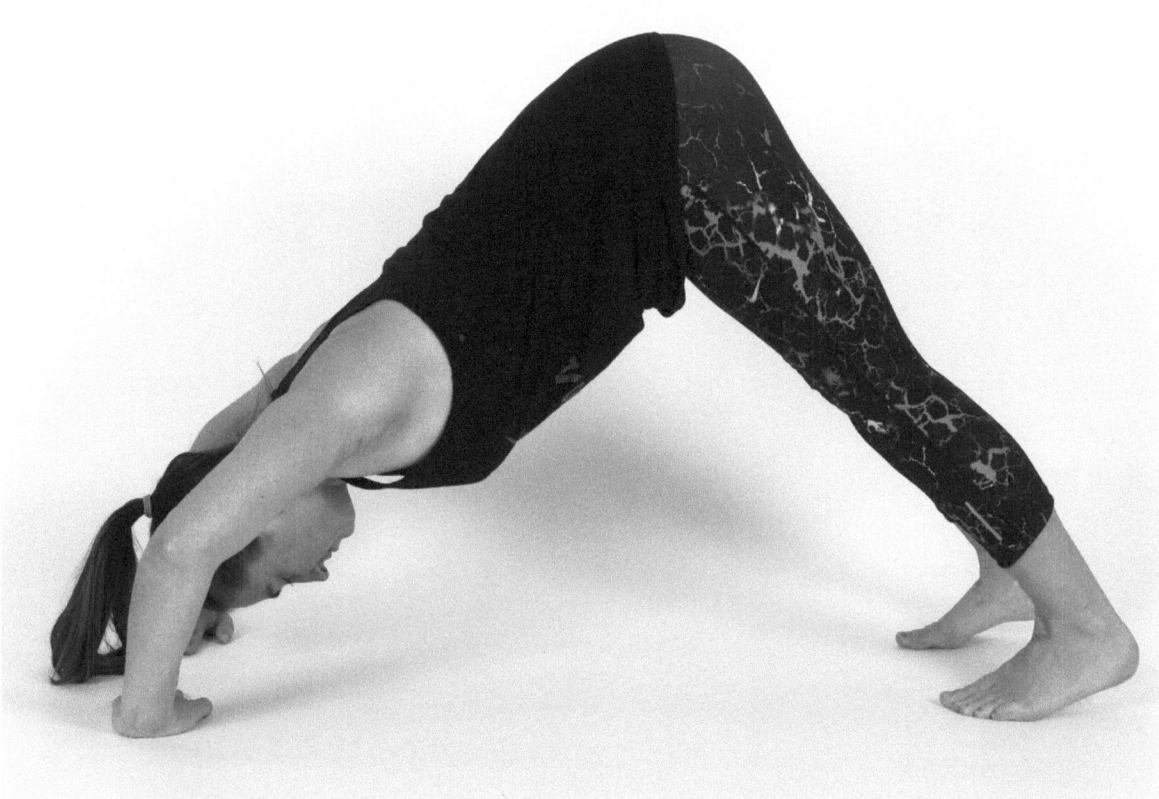

Getting yourself into the a downward dog position as in the picture, turn the hands in towards each other and keep the weight in the upper body and shoulders, now use the arms to press up in this position – try lowering the head down to the mat and pushing back up. You should attempt to achieve as many 'dips' as possible in 1 minute and repeat 3 sets with 20 second rests

Press-ups

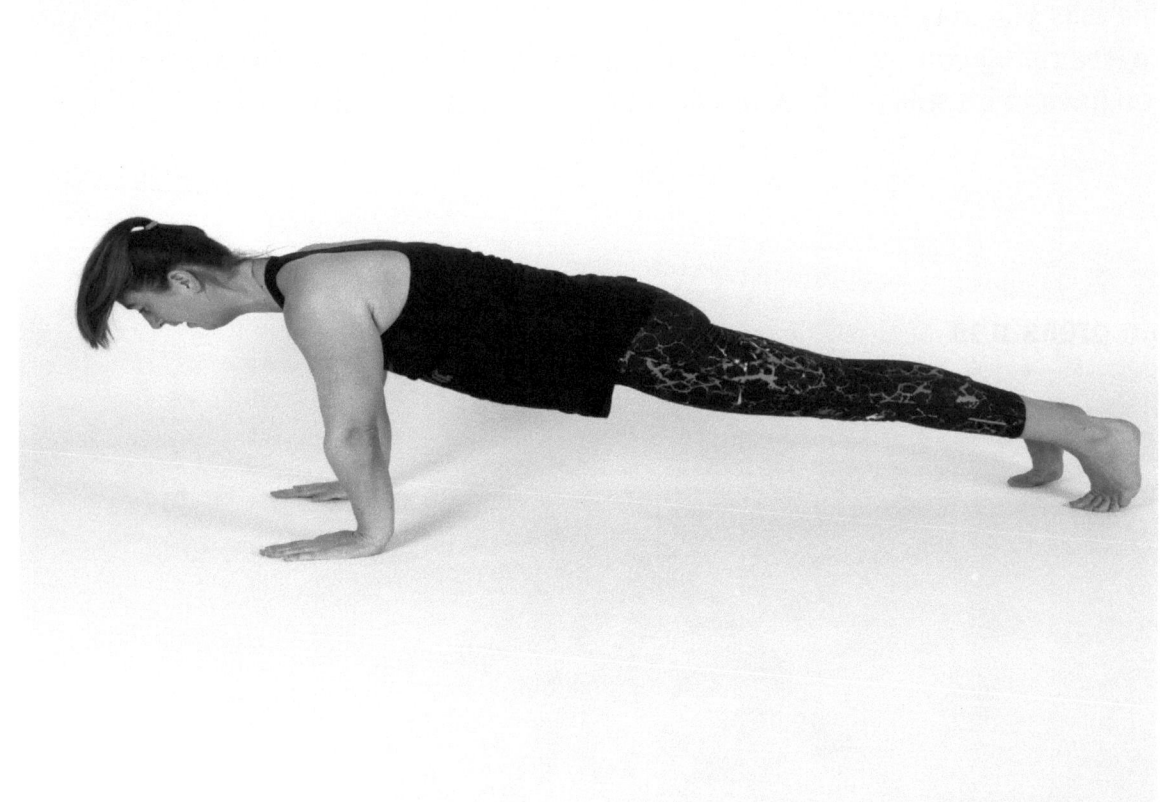

Standard press-ups not only work the shoulders, triceps and biceps but will strengthen the core too! Try sets of 10 building to 15 with 30 seconds rest in between
There is no need to use weights and this can be done anywhere!

- Press-ups can be a challenge for those with weak shoulders and arms, so try and build up your strength by adding one more each time – remember to keep the weight over the shoulders and wrists

Triceps dips plain and with leg

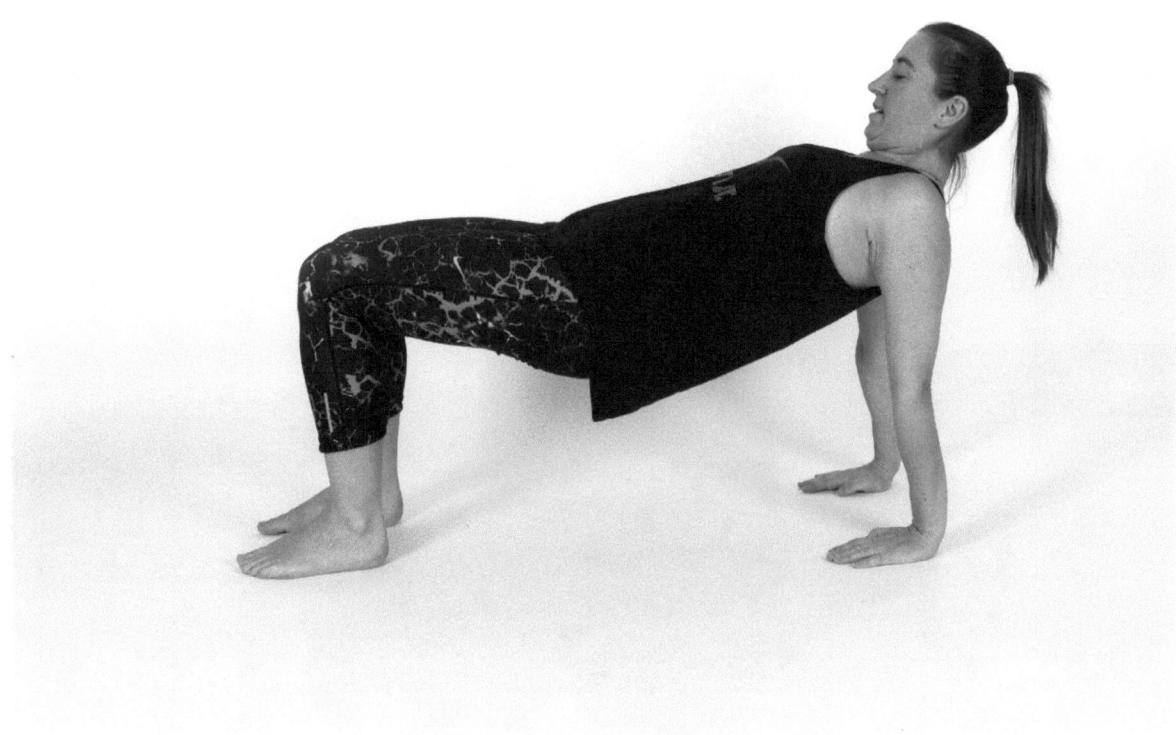

Set up the triceps dip making sure the shoulders are over the wrists, dip only using the arms and not hips.
You can also do these with a step, a yoga block – or at the bottom of your stairs.

Doing sets (as many as you can with one count for lower and one count for straitening) for 30 seconds and then add the leg raise: 15 seconds on each leg.

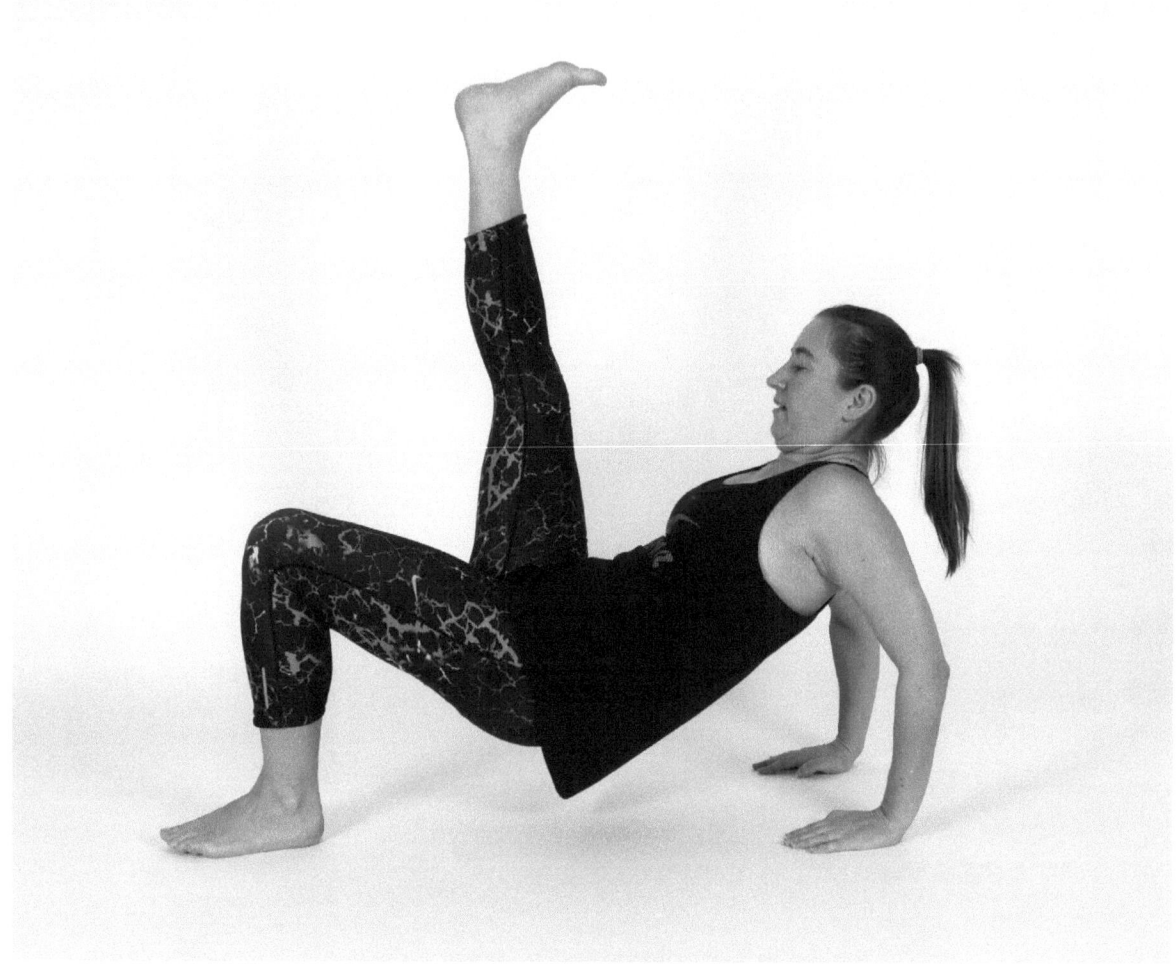

Again, short breaks to release the stress on the wrists if you have weaker wrists, you will find that strengthening the wrists doing these exercises will reduce the risk of breakage – the number one learner injury!!!

Core –

As important as leg strength is core strength. A strong core holds balance there is less chance of falling if core is strong, if you catch an edge you can use a the core to stabilize yourself. All these core exercises should be done daily before and during your trip.

I recommend that you perform at least 16 of each exercise (8 times on each side) and repeat the complete set twice.

Basic Crunches

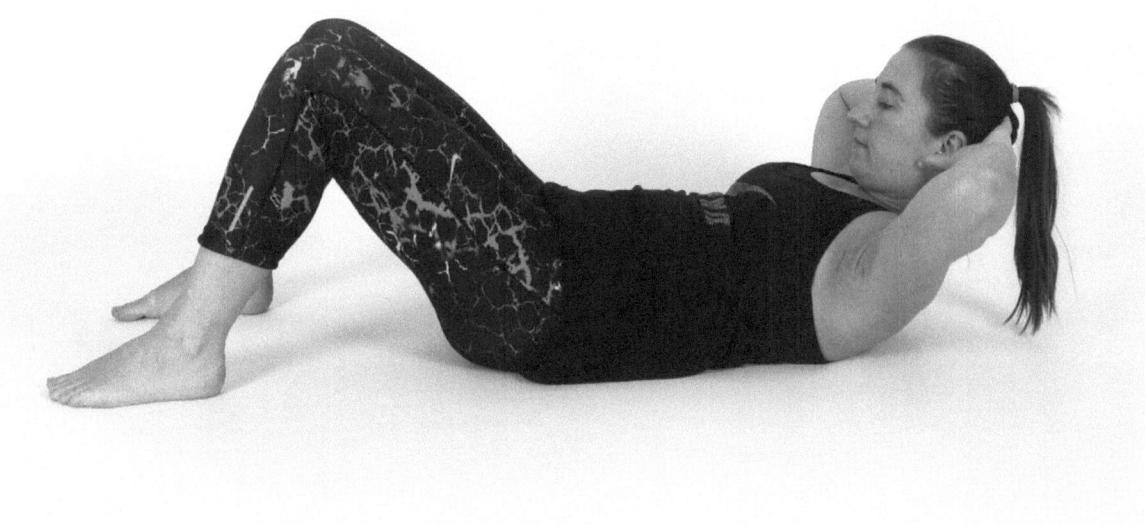

Set up for the basic crunch: lying on the back, feet shoulder width apart, flat on the floor. Place the hands behind the head or at the ears. Try to push the lower spine into the floor and keep the hips still.

Performing a basic crunch means lifting the head and shoulders off the floor to the shoulder blades (or bra strap for a woman). Breathing out on the way up and in in the way back down.

Oblique heel reach

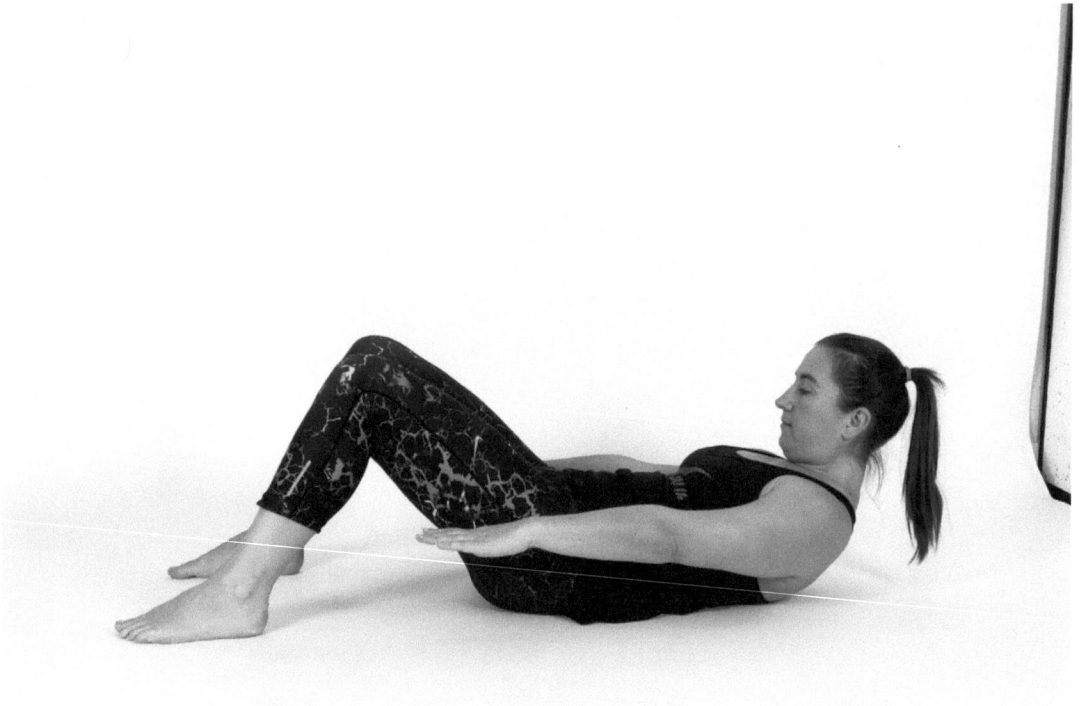

Stay up in the basic crunch and stretch the arm out to the sides of the body.

Next, reach the hand towards the right heel, bring it back to centre and then towards the left heel an Next, reach the hand towards the right heel, bring it back to centre and then towards the left heel and repeat going from left to right.

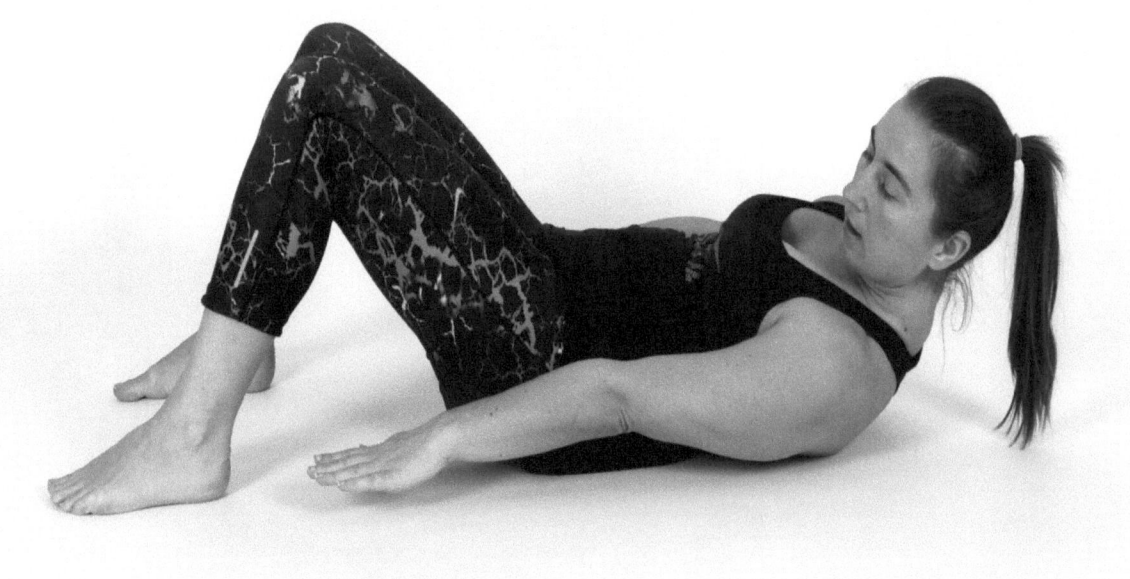

- If you are feeling tension in the neck because of a lack of core strength lower the head to begin with or have 10 seconds rest in between sets

Straight leg crunches with leg lifts

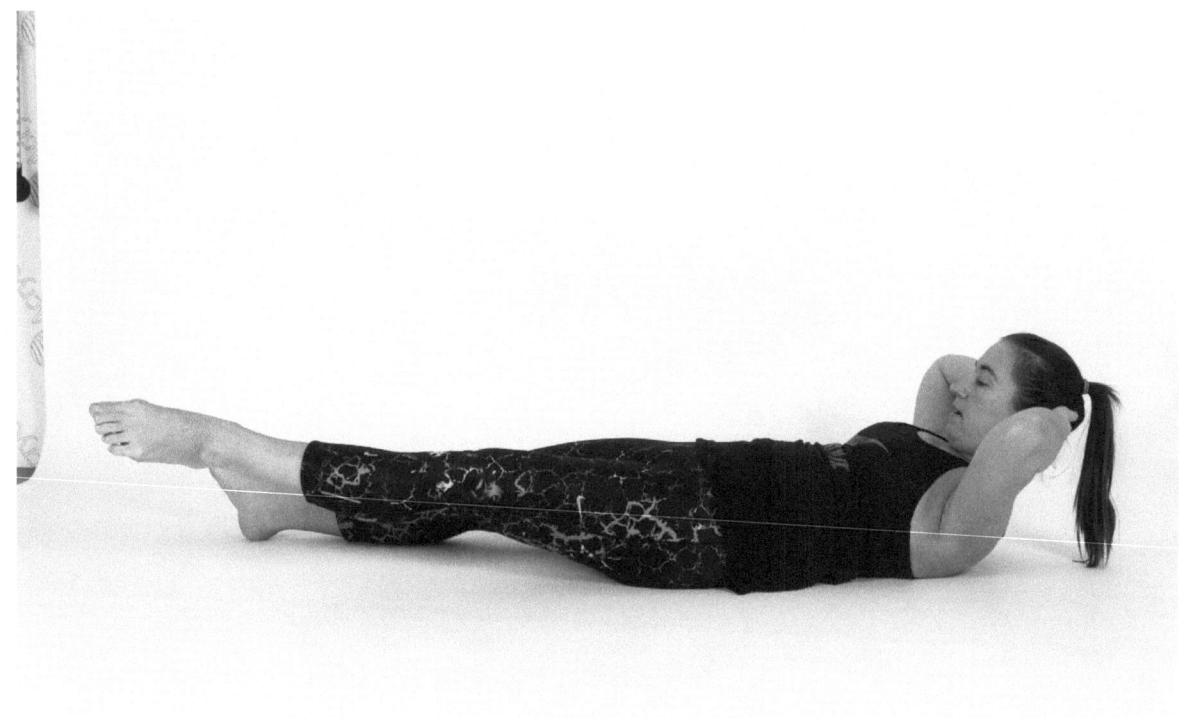

Now perform the basic crunch but with legs stretched out and slightly wider than shoulder width, after 8 plain crunches with the legs straight, raise each leg a few inches off the ground with the crunch 4 times each side:

- *Don't forget to breathe!!!!*
- *Breath out on the effort (crunching) and in on the recovery (lowering)*

The Hundred

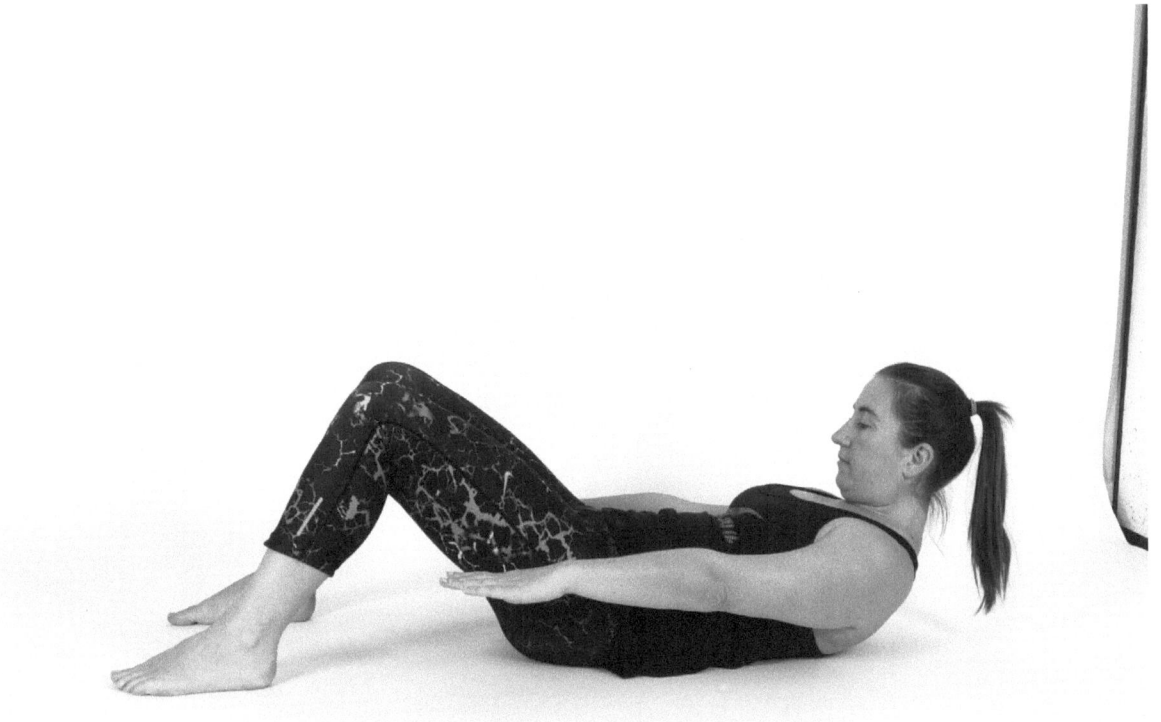

The hundred is a Pilates exercise, bringing yourself up to a stretched arm crunch beat the arms up and down with even beats (keep arms straight) as you beat breath in for 5 counts and out for 5 counts 10 times (totaling 100)

Rest, repeat section but add a 1 min plank instead of the 100.

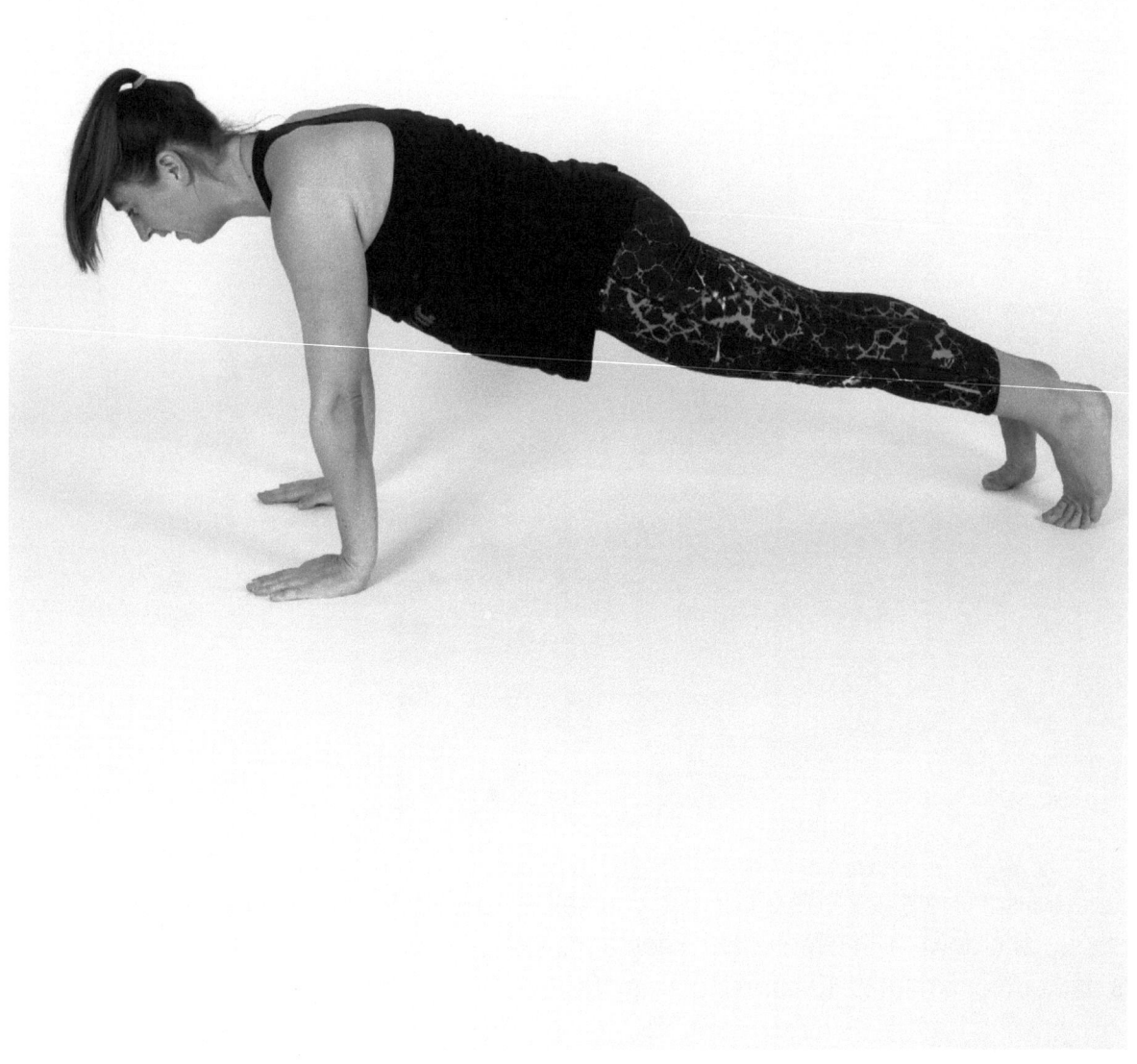

Plank – basic plank should be held for a minimum of one minute, keep the body in a straight line and shoulders over wrists. You should try to add an extra 10 seconds each time you do these – see how many minutes you can do after 1 month!

Stretches – it is important to stretch out at the end of an exercise session, stretching will lengthen the muscles and get rid of any lactic acid build up. Stretching in snowboarding is important to improve your flexibility so that your body and muscles can cope with the positions you may put it into without causing injury.

Most of these stretches are from my Yoga practice, but I will explain them without the use of yoga terminology.

Parallel Legs Forward Bend

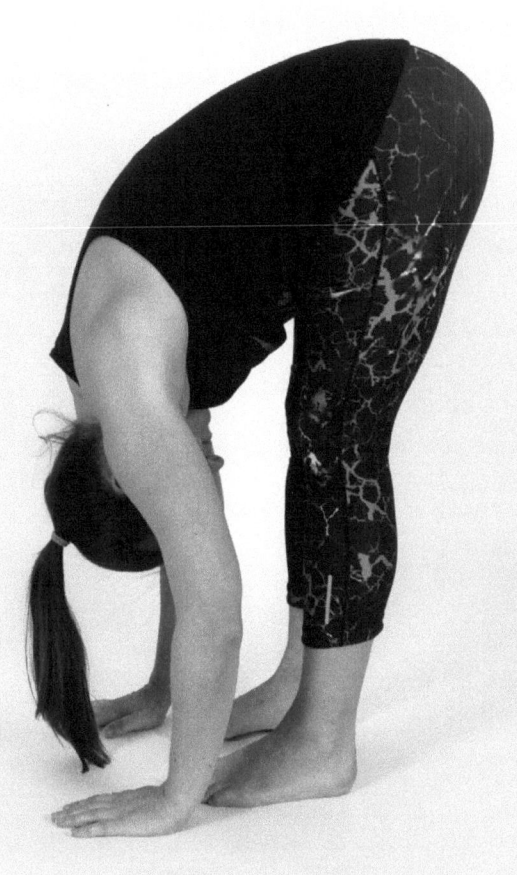

Standing with your feet together and facing forward roll down through the spine until you go as far as you can – aim to improve the stretch each time you perform it, building up to being able to pull the chest into the thigh and hold the arms behind the ankle. Hold

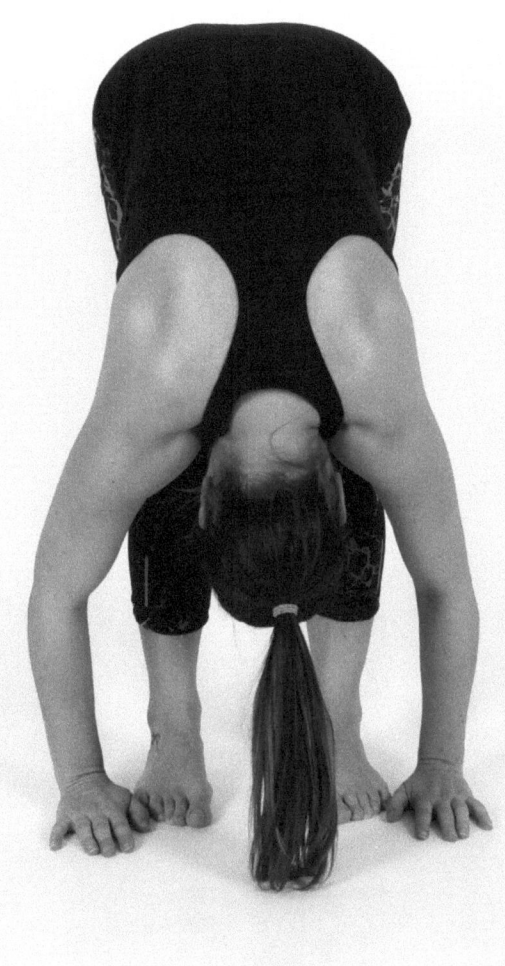

Stretching the hamstrings this will also add strength to the lower back. Hold for 5 deep in and out breathes

Extended side stretch

Set up this position by taking a wide leg stance and then lowering the weight onto one side by bending the knee into a right angle, keeping the knee over the toe reach the top arm as far away as you can to stretch the side of the body and add strength into the legs, hold for 5 deep in and out breaths.

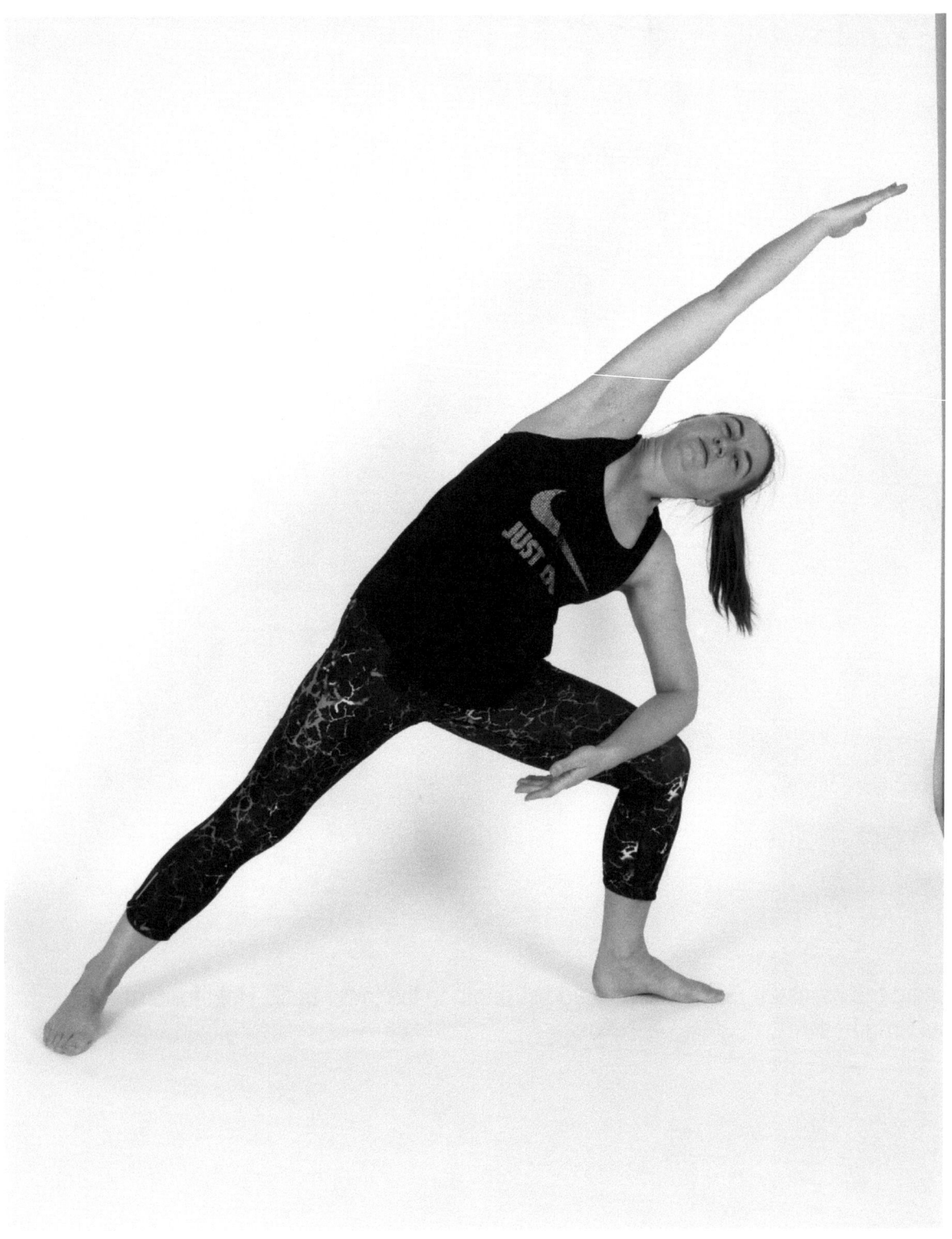

Hip flexor

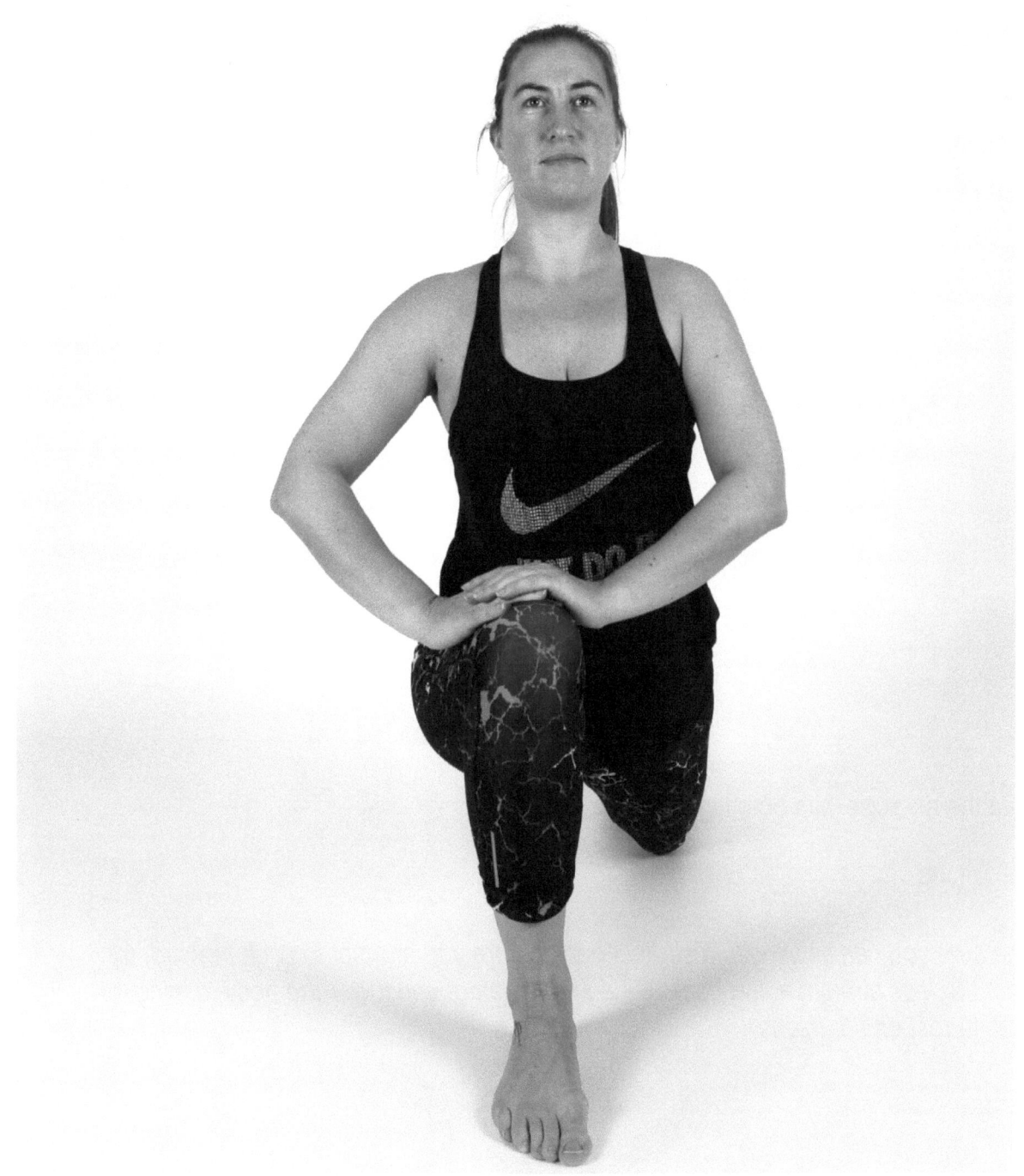

Seated parallel

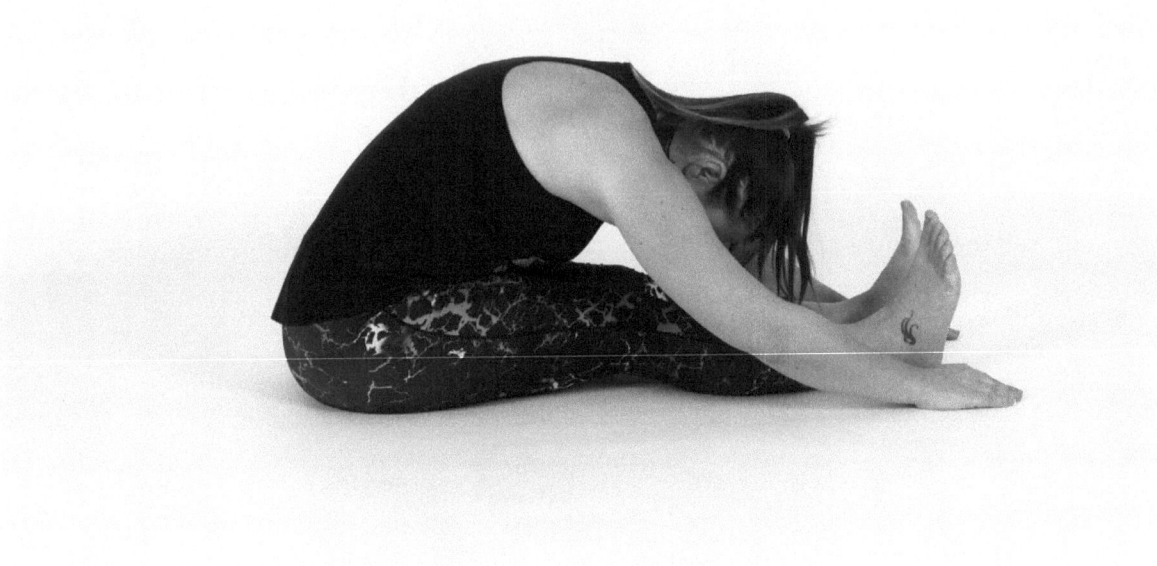

Repeat the exercise with both legs straight.

- Make sure you can sit up with a straight back before you attempt to pitch forward, try and get the legs straight at the back of the knees before you lower the body, aiming for the ribs to rest on the thighs

Seated one leg

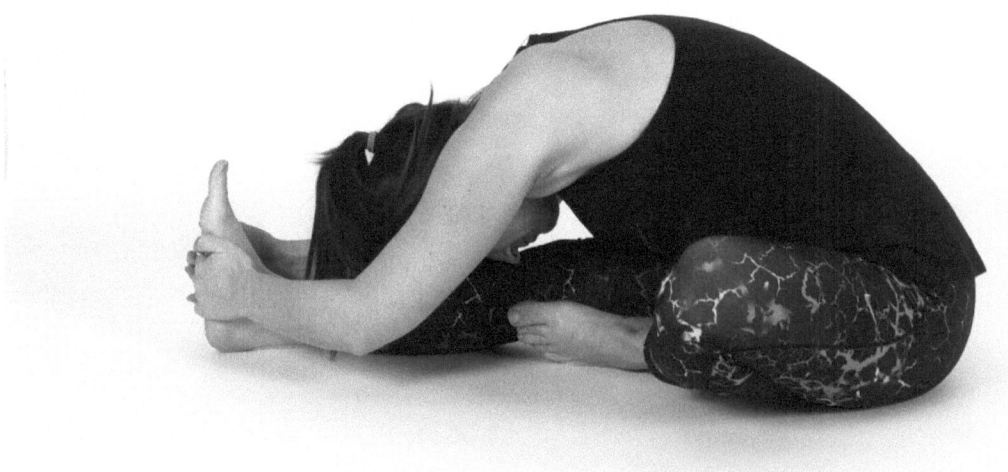

Sit upright with the legs straight out in front of you. Bring the right leg in with foot in line with opposite knee, now stretch forward over the left leg, keeping the gaze forward think about bringing the ribs to the thighs. Hold for 5 deep in and out breathes. Repeat on other leg.

As well as the training programme I have devised a pre slope warm up that should be performed on waking, before you eat and before you go on the slopes for the day

Pre slope warm up

Sun salute

Sun salute is the basic warm up sequence used in Yoga practice, it can be used as a daily warm up and will not only warm all the major muscle groups but done without stops can also raise the heart beat. Try to flow from one position to the next using in and out breaths. This is using the principles of Ashtanga Yoga and if unsure of how the positions link together please watch my YouTube instruction or use the getfitSnow app

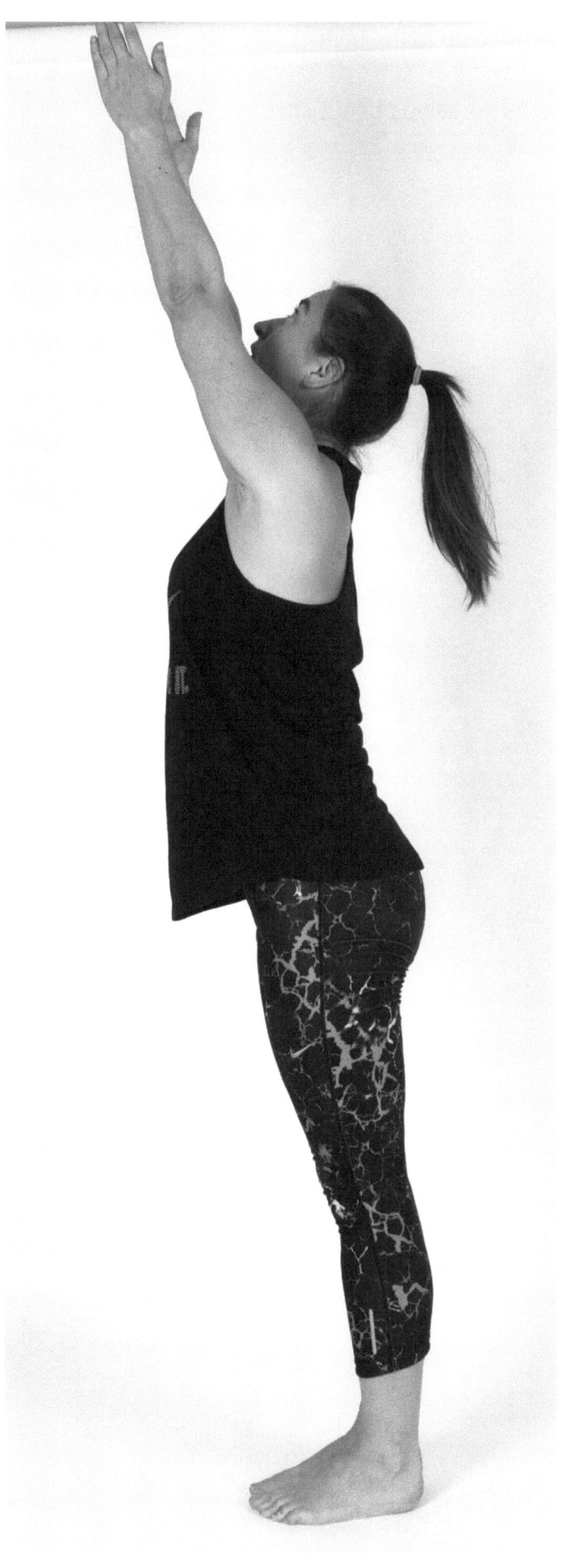

Sun Salutation A

Starting at the end of the mat with your feet shoulder width apart, tummy sucked in and shoulders down. Inhale on the movement of the arms

Raise your arms above your head, taking the gaze up to the hands

Lower the body and reach for the toes, going as far as you can. Exhale

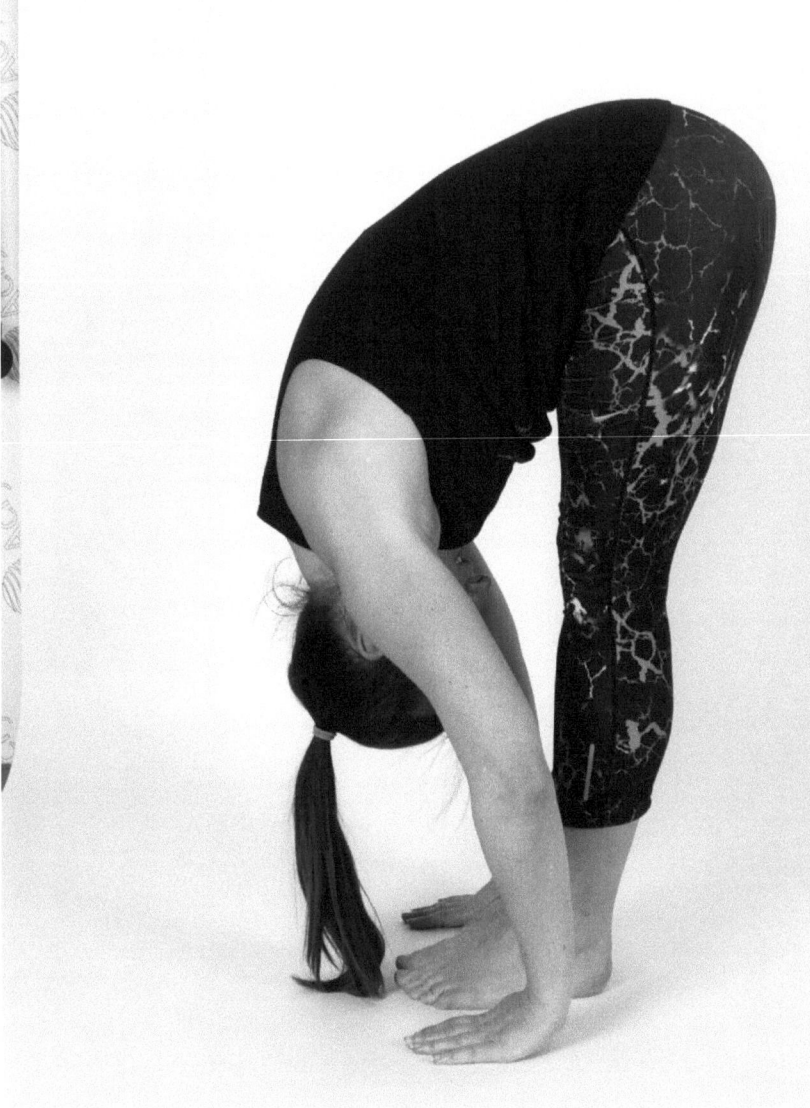

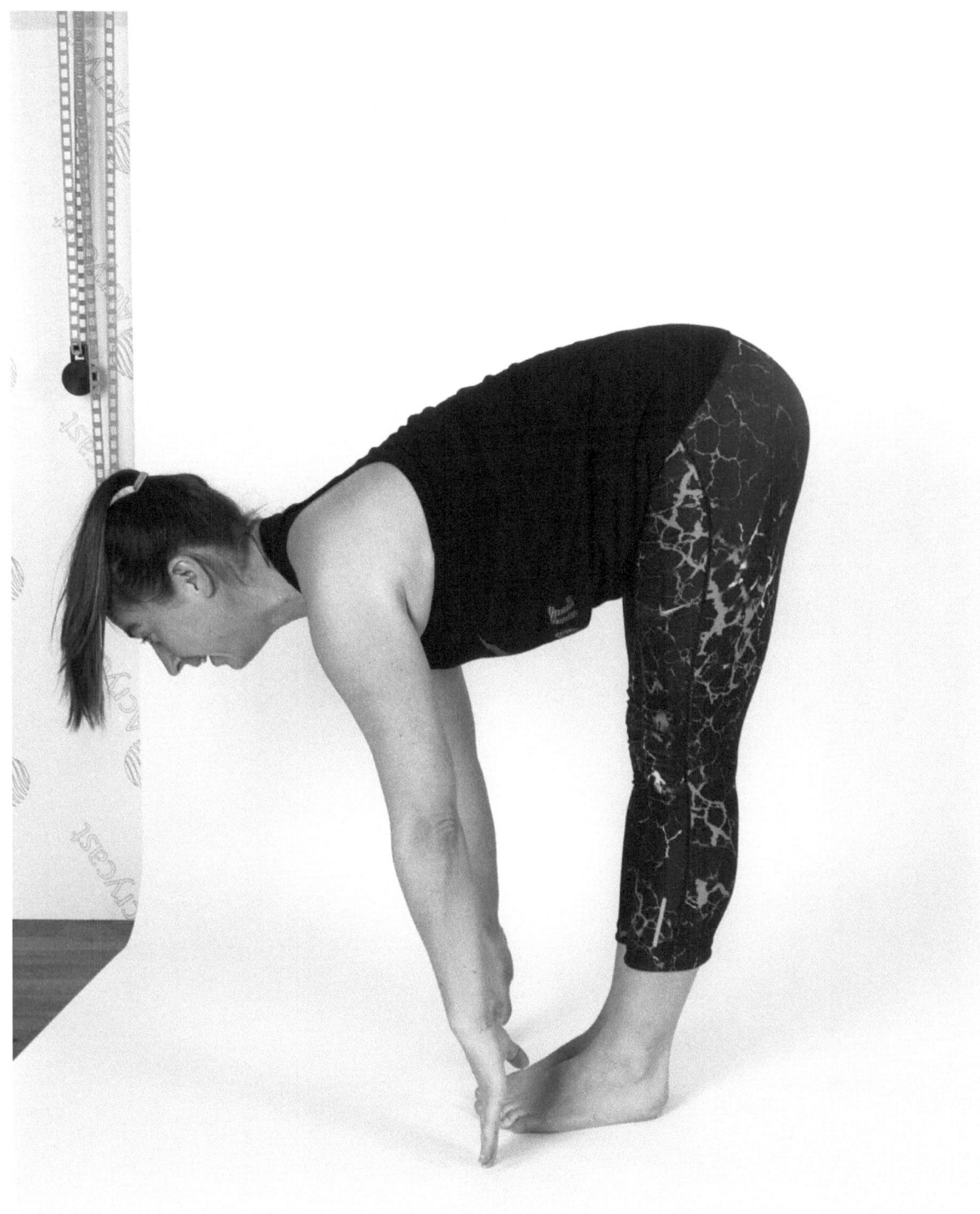

Raise the head and lengthen out the back. Inhale.

Exhale, Lower the head again and bend the knees so that you can place the hands flat on the floor either side of the feet, keeping them under the shoulders

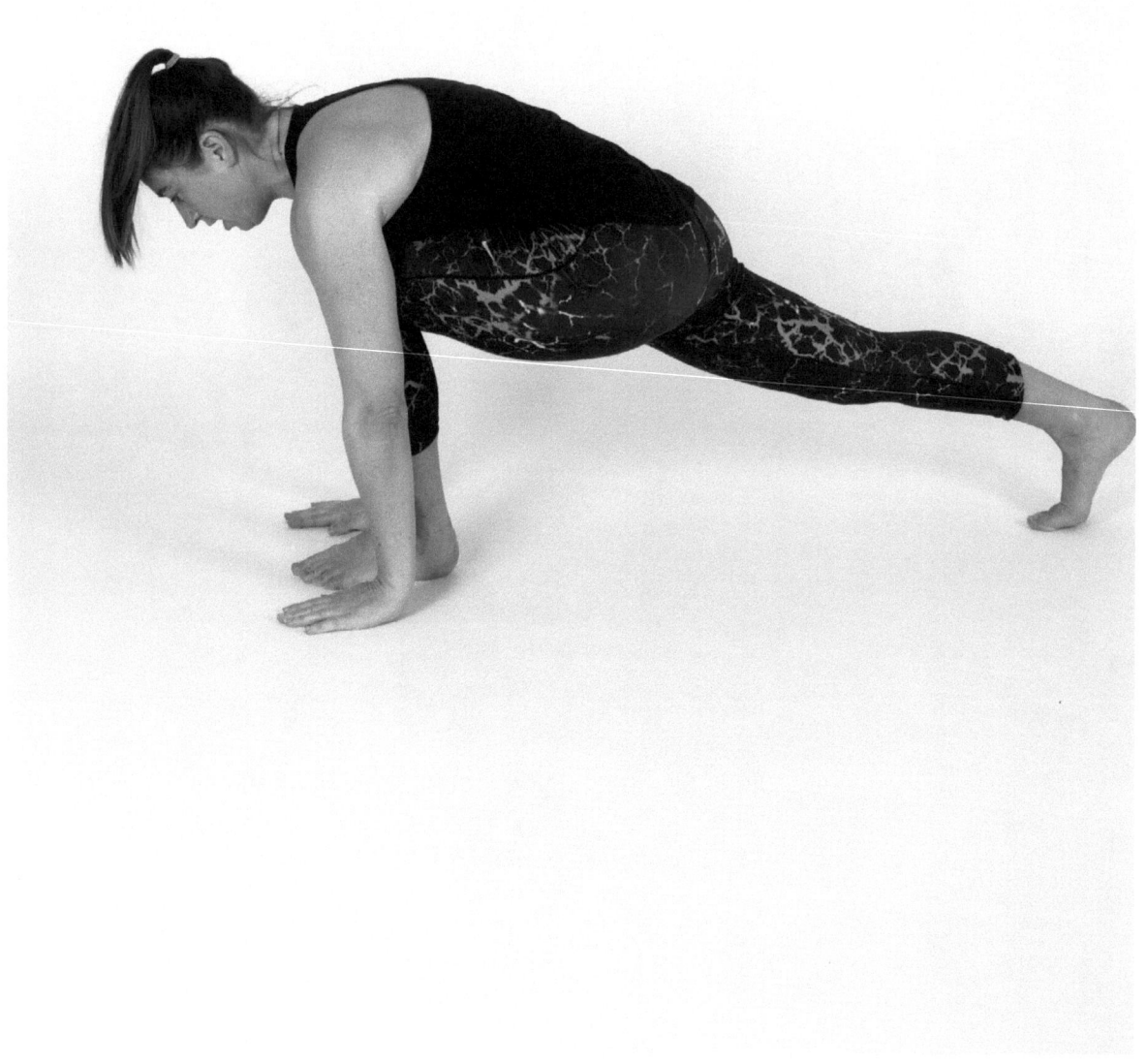

Take the right foot back, keeping it straight with no bend in the knee.

Take the left foot back to join the right foot so you are in the plank position, keeping the weight over the shoulders and hands.

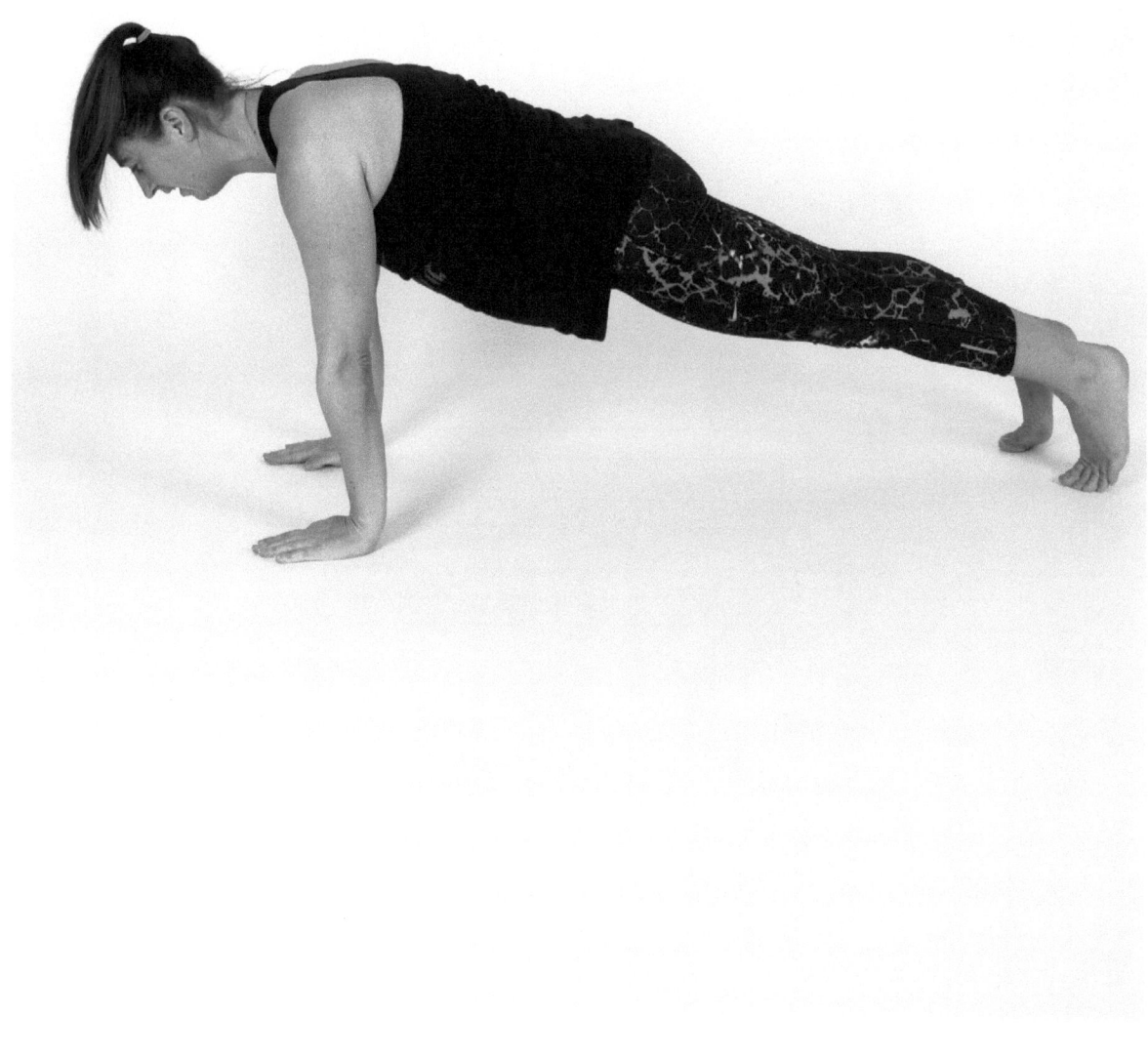

Lower the body down to keeping the elbows in

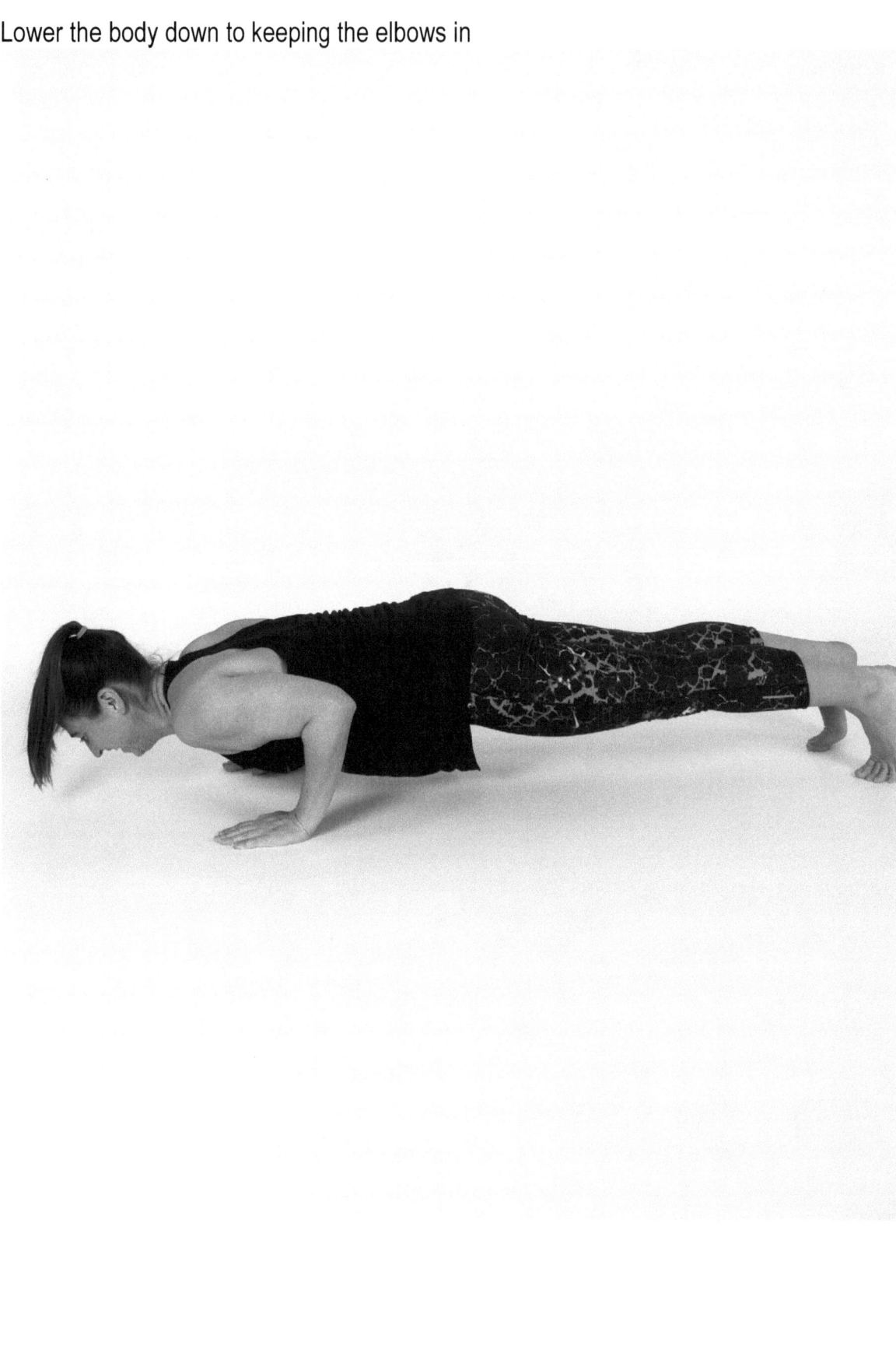

Bring the head and back up into the cobra pose, keep the shoulder blades drawn down the back

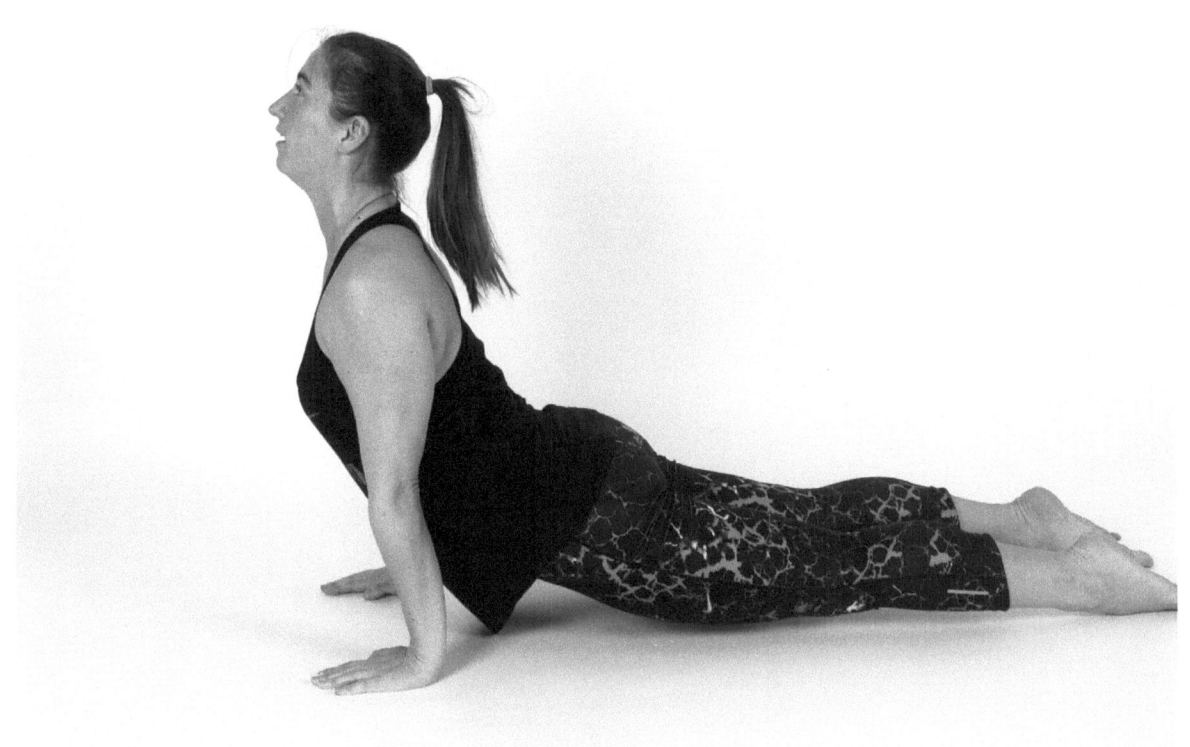

Tuck the toes in and push the bottom up so you are in the downward dog position
HOLD the downward dog for 5 deep in and out breaths

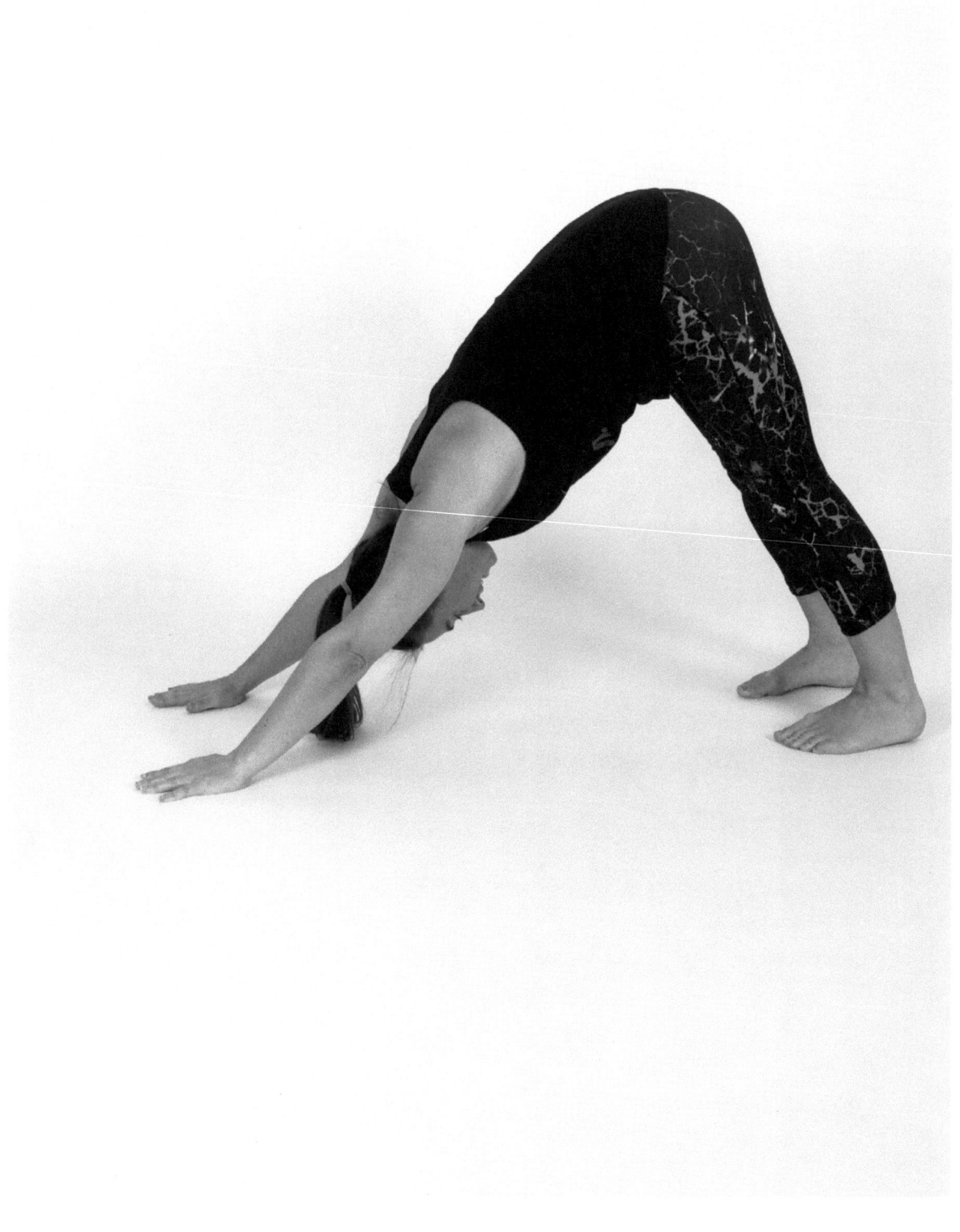

Take the gaze to the hands; bring the left leg and foot back into the space between the hands.

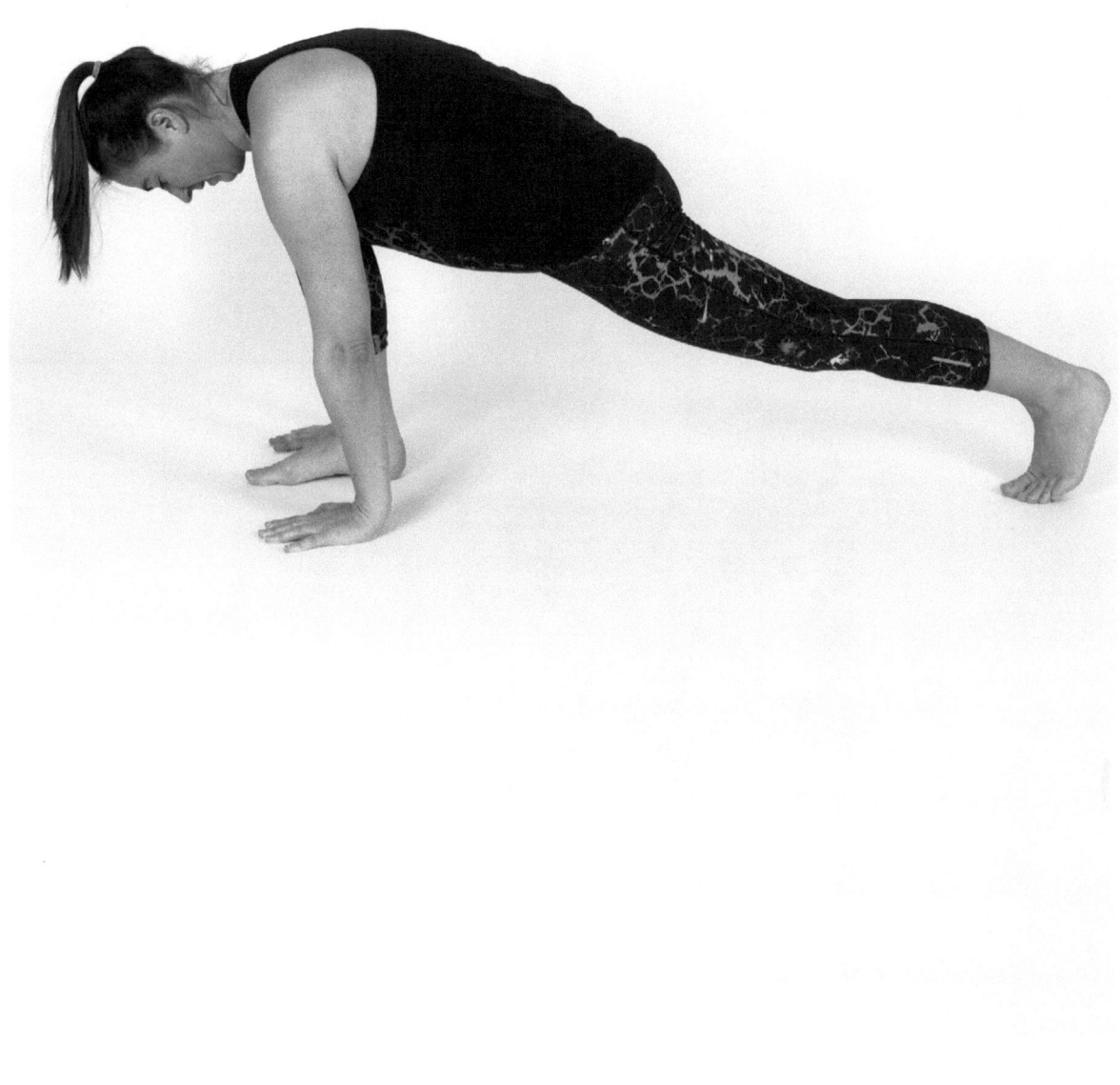

Bring the other foot in.

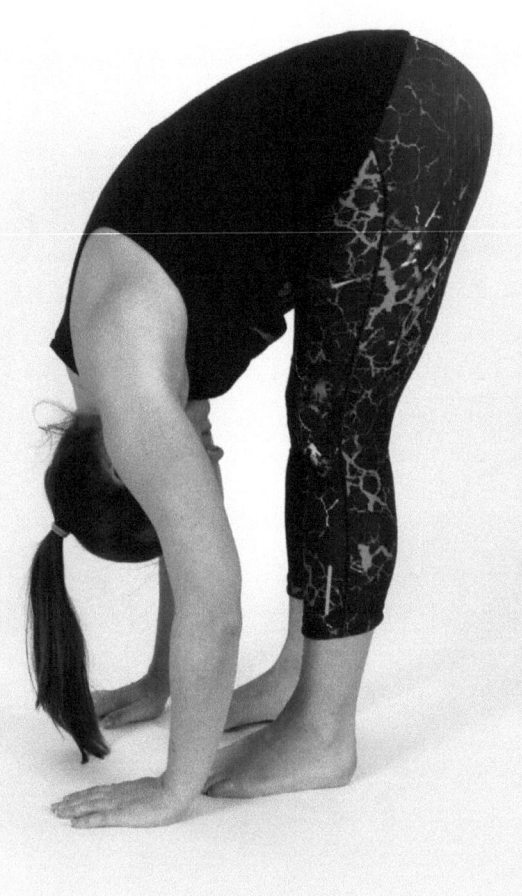

Inhale, Straighten up bringing the head over the head, and then slowly lower the arms to bring yourself back to the starting position. Exhale

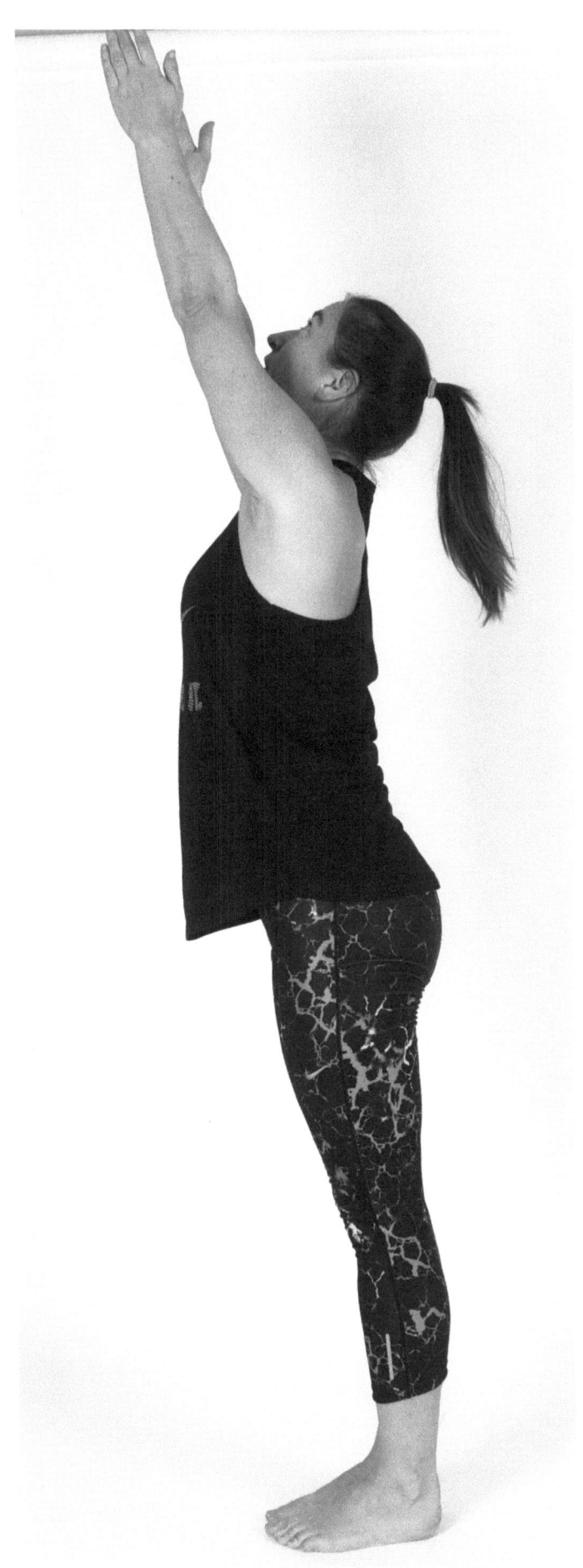

Core section (pre slope warm up)

Crunches

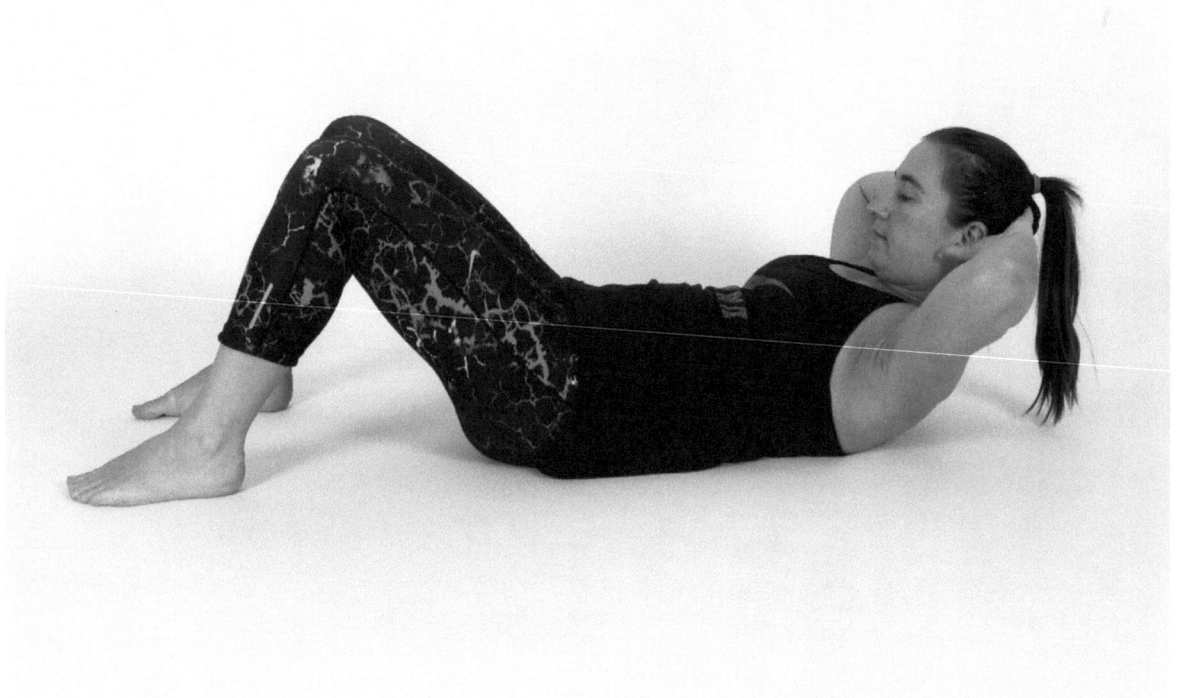

Set up for the basic crunch: lying on the back, feet shoulder width apart, flat on the floor. Place the hands behind the head or at the ears. Try to push the lower spine into the floor and keep the hips still.
Performing a basic crunch means lifting the head and shoulders off the floor to the shoulder blades (or bra strap for a woman). Breathing out on the way up and in in the way back down.

Oblique heel reach

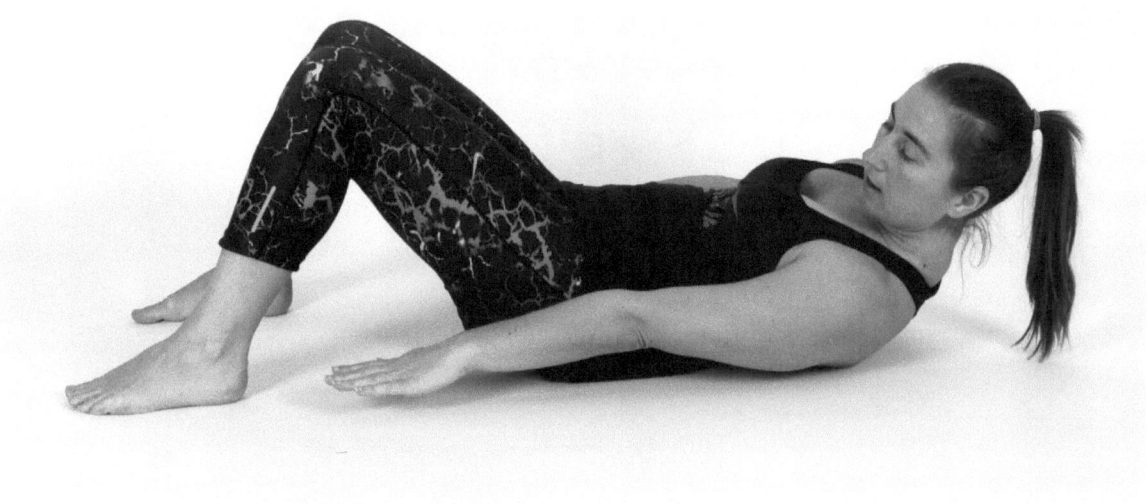

Stay up in the basic crunch and stretch the arm out to the sides of the body.

Now reach the hand towards the right heel, bring it back to centre and then towards the left heel and repeat.

Straight leg crunches with leg lifts

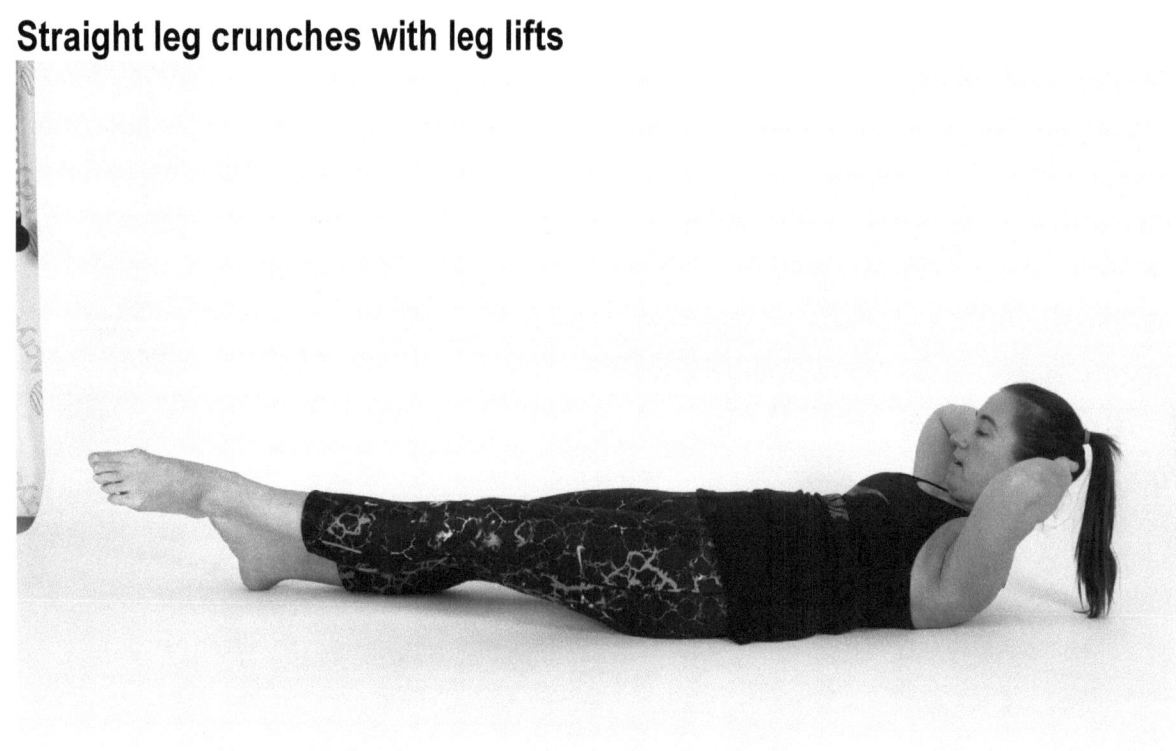

Now perform the basic crunch but with legs stretched out and slightly wider than shoulder width, after 8 plain raise each leg with the crunch 4 times each side:

Lift each leg with each crunch

The Hundred

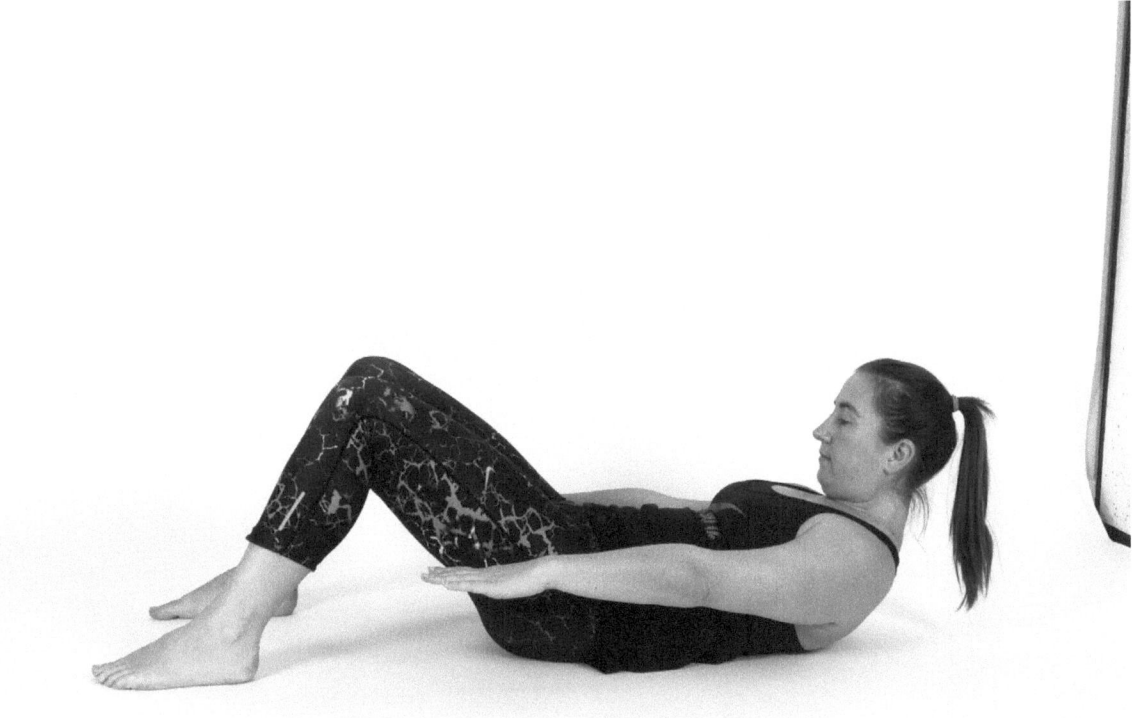

The hundred is a Pilates exercise, bringing yourself up to a stretched arm crunch beat the arms up and down with even beats (keep arms straight) as you beat breath in for 5 counts and out for 5 counts 10 times (totaling 100)

Rest, repeat section but add a 1 min plank instead of the 100.

Warrior 1

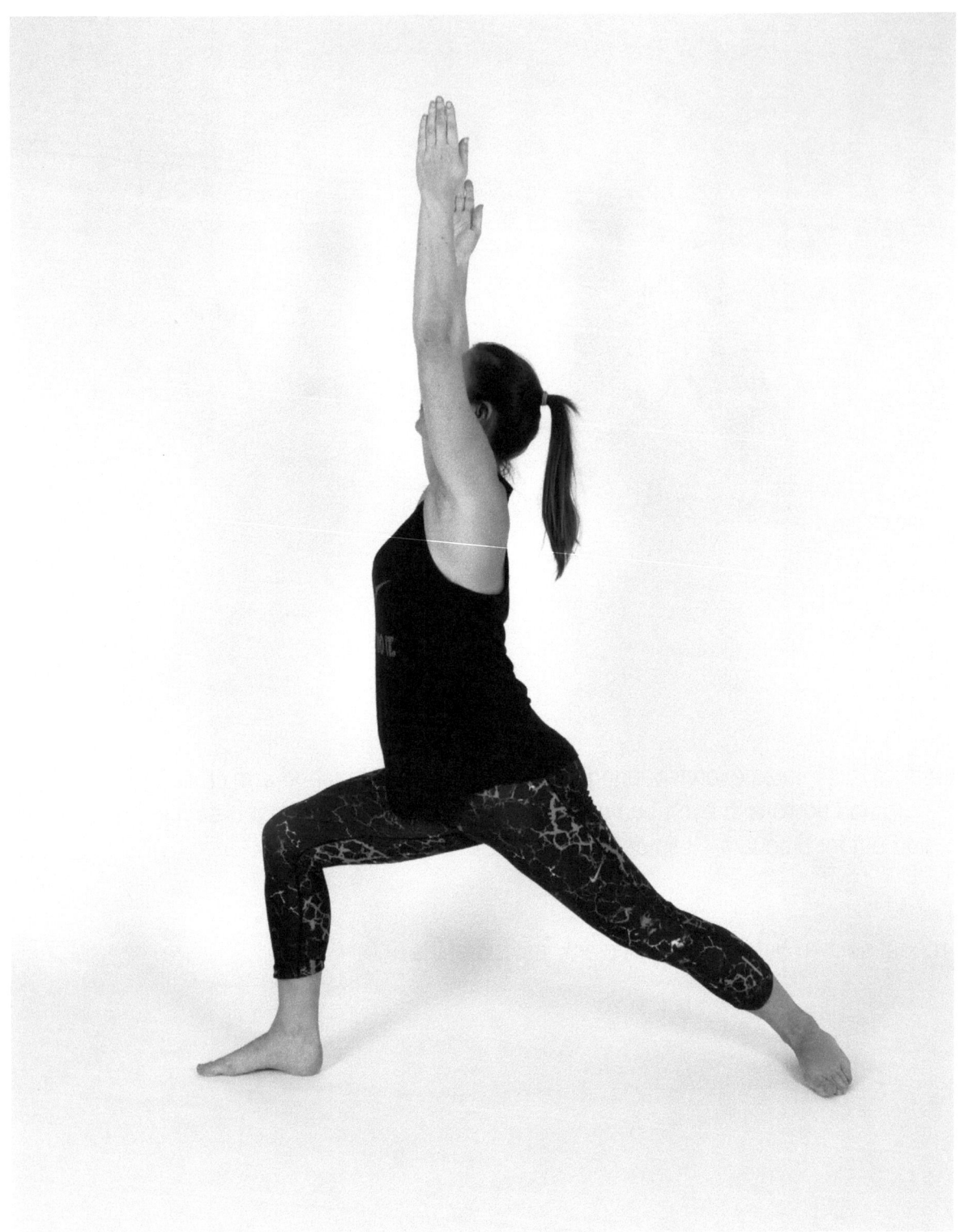

Hold this posture to develop strength in the legs for 5 inhale and exhales

Exhale into the next posture:
Warrior 2

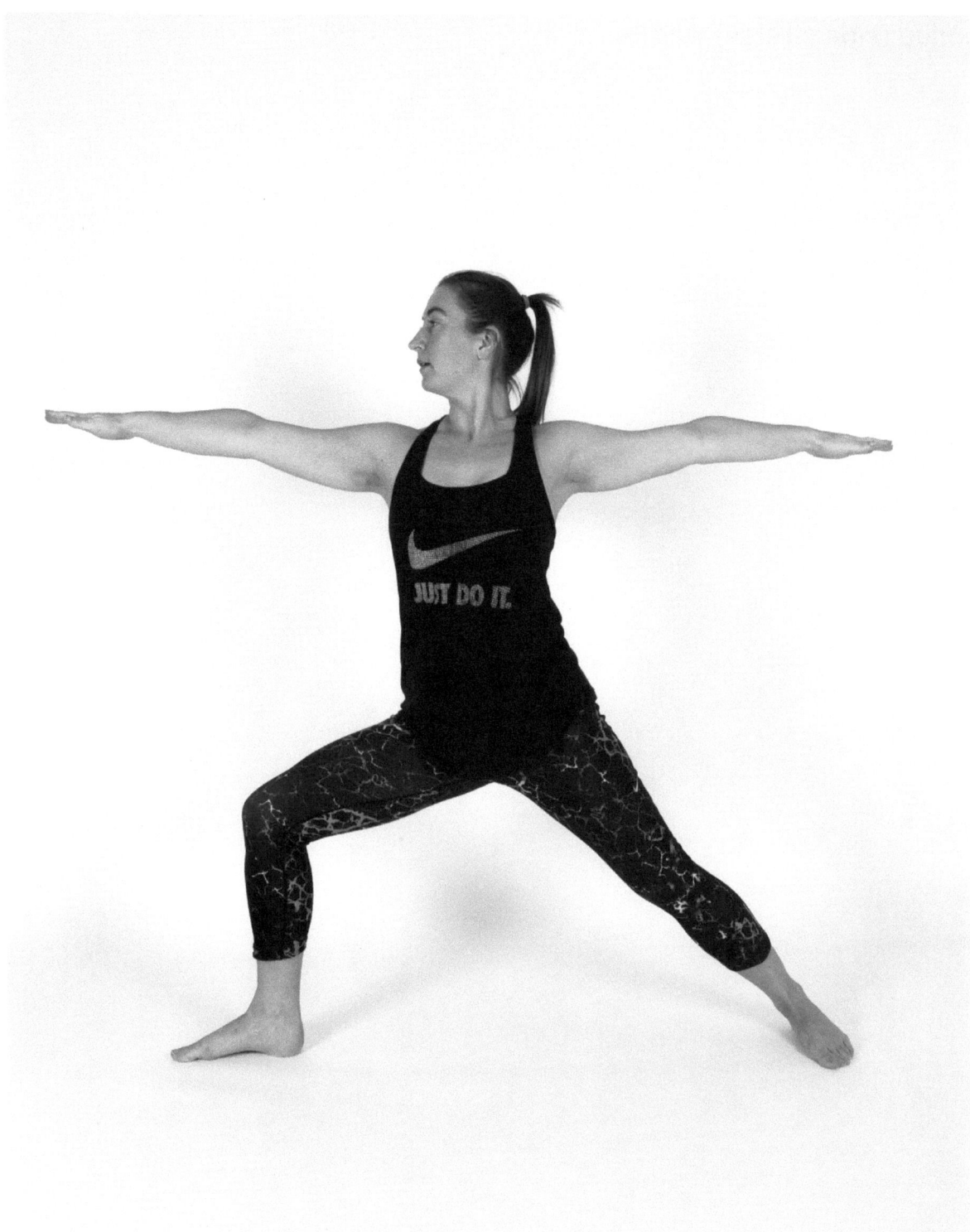

Start with a wide leg stance, then turn out the left (front) foot and turn in the right (back) foot. Bend the knee over the front foot, making sure you have knee over toe but that you can still see your foot, do not over stretch this. Raise the arms to shoulder height and take gaze over the front arm. Hold.

Extended (side stretch) warrior

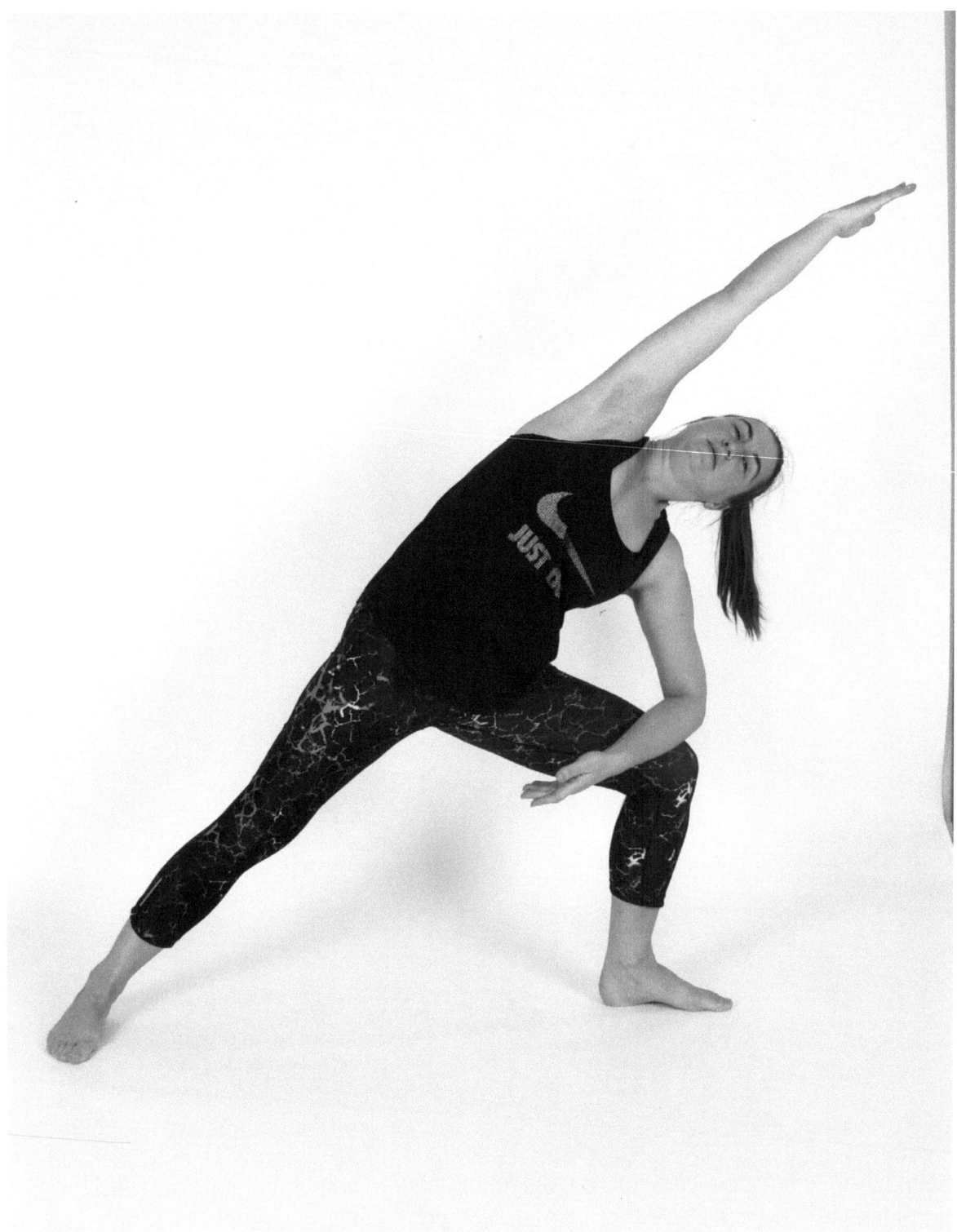

To extend the warrior pose when you are more flexible lower the front arm in line with the front foot and raise back arm up, take the gaze up to the top arm.

Quad and Hip flexor stretch

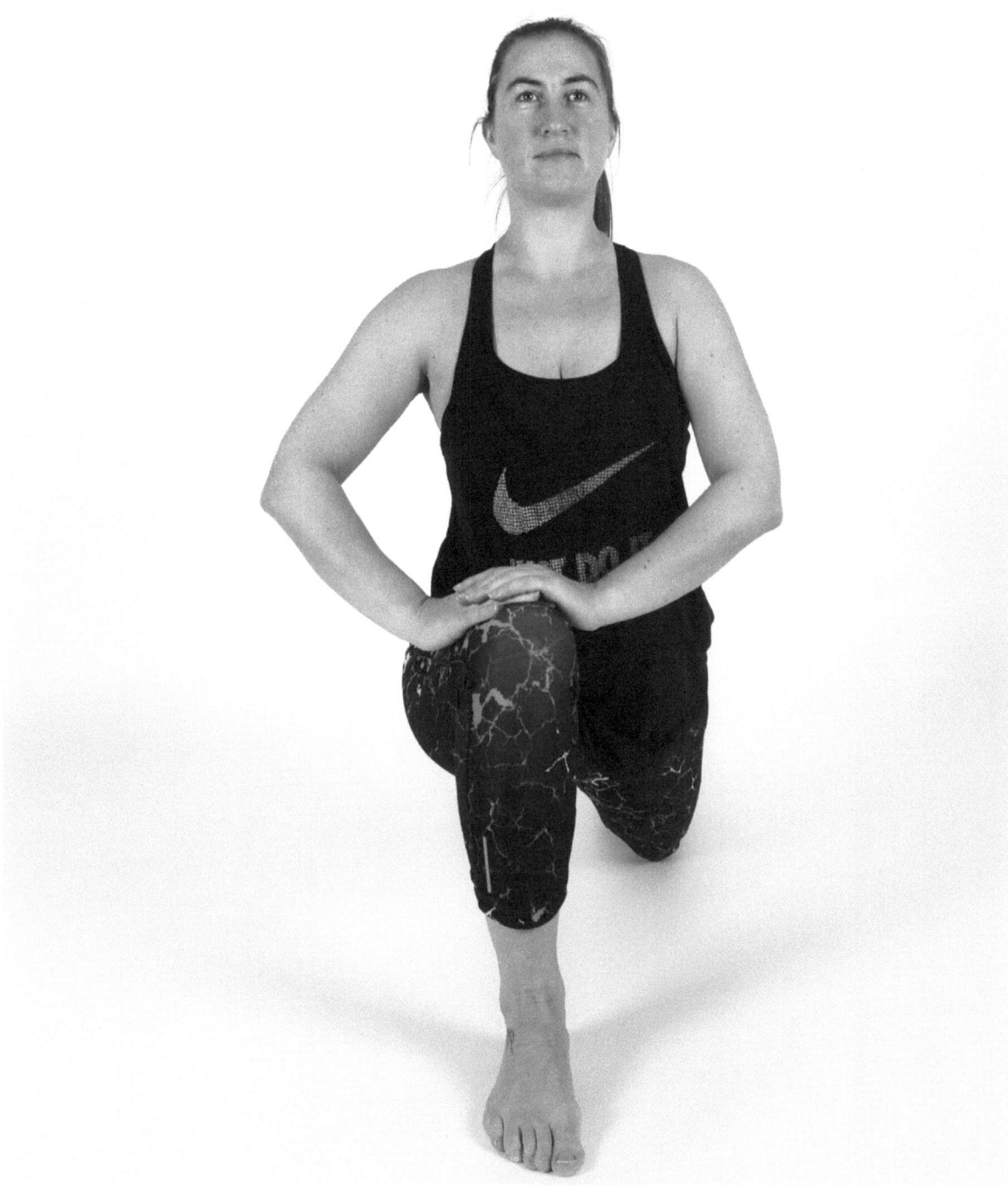

Place the front leg on the floor at a right angle, with the back knee on the floor, gently push into the hip flexor to stretch out, hold for 20 seconds, and repeat on both sides Push a little further than previous times to extend the stretch into your quads

Post slope stretch

It is important to stretch after your daily session – preferably before you head to après!!!

Some of these stretches, warrior, triangle and a basic quad stretch can be done at the bottom of the slopes in your kit, or ideal perform the following before your shower or sauna.

Parallel

Wide leg stretch, A and B

Extended side stretch

Hip flexor

That concludes the GetFit for snowboarding workouts, I hope they have given you some ideas and you can either follow them explicitly or adapt them to suit your needs.

For further information and new stretches and training ideas please go to
www.getfitsnow.co.uk
http://getfitsnow.blogspot.co.uk/

Or buy the app from the app store – coming soon!

And happy, safe boarding!

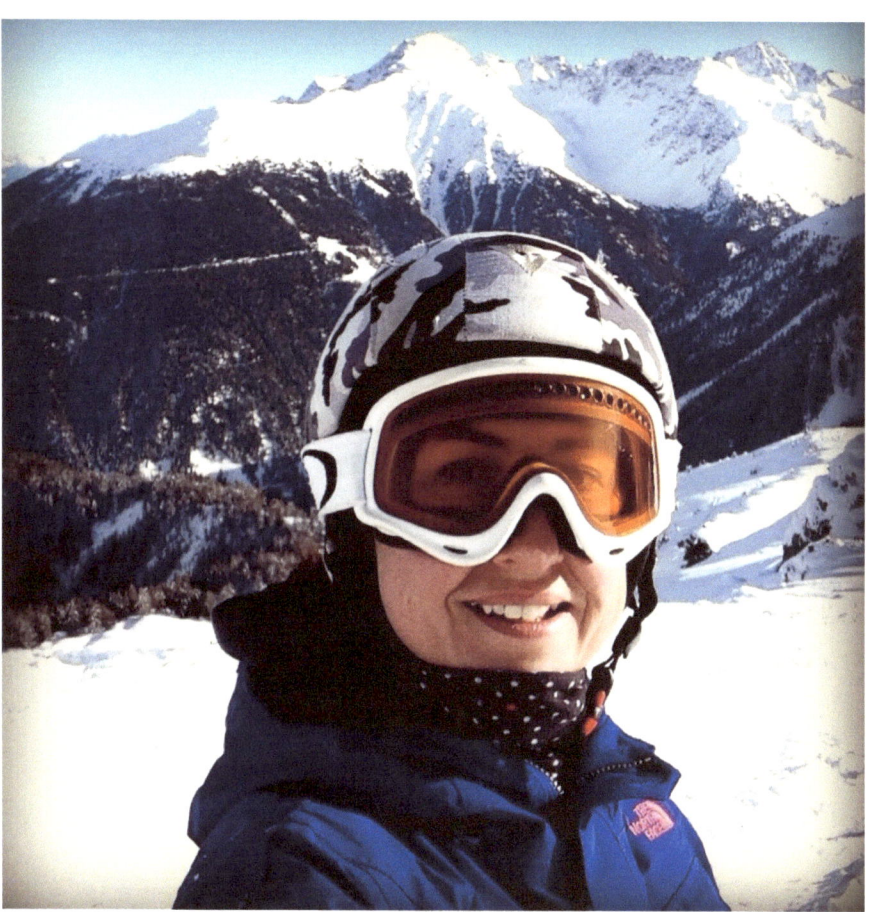

www.ingramcontent.com/pod-product-compliance
Lightning Source LLC
Chambersburg PA
CBHW041518280526

45792CB00004B/1293